Veröffentlichungen aus der
Geomedizinischen Forschungsstelle
(Leiter: Professor Dr. med. Helmut J. Jusatz)
der Heidelberger Akademie der Wissenschaften

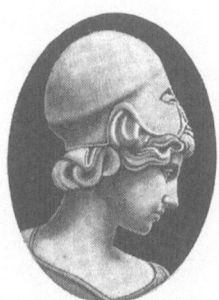

Supplement zu den Sitzungsberichten der
Mathematisch-naturwissenschaftlichen Klasse
Jahrgang 1982

Bernhard M. Thimm

Brucellosis

Distribution in Man, Domestic and Wild Animals

Foreword by Wilhelm Wundt

With 3 coloured Map Plates
of Europe, Africa and America
and 2 Figures

Submitted to the Meeting of 25 April, 1981
by Richard Haas

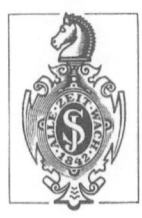

Springer-Verlag
Berlin Heidelberg GmbH   1982

Dr. med. vet. Bernhard M. Thimm

Fachtierarzt für Tropenveterinärmedizin,
Leiter der Krankenhaushygiene der Universität Ulm
– Klinikum –, Steinhövelstraße 9
D-7900 Ulm

Dr. med. habil. Wilhelm Wundt

o. Prof. und Direktor des Instituts für Hygiene und Med.
Mikrobiologie der Fakultät für Klinische Medizin Mann-
heim der Universität Heidelberg, Theodor-Kutzer-Ufer,
D-6800 Mannheim 1

English Translation by

J. A. Hellen, M. A. (Oxon.), Dr. phil. (Bonn)
and Mrs. I. F. Hellen
Newcastle upon Tyne

CIP-Kurztitelaufnahme der Deutschen Bibliothek

Thimm, Bernhard M.;
Brucellosis : distribution in man, domestic and wild animals / Bernhard M. Thimm. With a
foreword by Wilhelm Wundt. Submitted to the meeting of 25 April, 1981 by Richard Haas. –
Berlin ; Heidelberg ; New York : Springer, 1982.
   (Veröffentlichungen aus der Geomedizinischen Forschungsstelle der Heidelberger Akademie der Wissenschaften) (Supplement zu den Sitzungsberichten der Mathematisch-Naturwissenschaftlichen Klasse / [Heidelberger Akademie der Wissenschaften] ; Jg. 1982)

   ISBN 978-3-642-81762-5   ISBN 978-3-642-81760-1 (eBook)
   DOI 10.1007/978-3-642-81760-1
NE: Heidelberger Akademie der Wissenschaften / Mathematisch-Naturwissenschaftliche
Klasse: Sitzungsberichte der Mathematisch-Naturwissenschaftlichen Klasse / Supplement

2125/3140-543210

Foreword

The distribution of brucellosis in Europe and the Mediterranean area had been cartographically represented by Horst Habs as early as 1942. The case of brucellosis presented a particularly exciting task of relating the areas where the species *Brucella melitensis, B. abortus* and, to a lesser degree, even *B. suis,* occurred, to geographical and climatic data, which in turn condition certain agricultural structures and forms of animal husbandry. In the World Atlas of Diseases, edited by Ernst Rodenwaldt and Helmut J. Jusatz on behalf of the Heidelberg Academy of Sciences, W. Wundt then published maps in 1956 and 1961 depicting the distribution of brucellosis and its three species of causal agent − *B. melitensis, B. abortus* and *B. suis* in Europe and the world − based on the data available at the time.

As more than 20 years have passed since the appearance of these maps, the time seemed ripe for the compilation of new maps and the suggestion was immediately taken up by the Geomedical Research Unit. The realisation that data on the occurrence of brucellosis had been rather fragmentary in many parts of the world at the time of the publication of the World Atlas of Diseases, and that this situation had improved in at least some regions of the world, had been one of the reasons for attempting an up-to-date presentation of the situation. Compared with the time at which the first world map was drawn up, data on the occurrence of brucellosis in its different forms and its reservoirs of the causative agents in the animal kingdom, particularly in South America, have become much more numerous and more easily evaluable. So, too, from Africa more material has become available, including some on the natural foci existing there, with the result that it became necessary to compile new maps for these continents.

In North America and Europe the picture has changed. Intensive control measures in the U.S.A. and Canada have led to a considerable decline, and in some areas to the extermination, of this animal disease, which can cause numerous chronic and protracted diseases in man as well. In Europe it was mainly the states of the northern and central European areas which succeeded in achieving the extermination or at least the regression of brucellosis. (The original plan to present the conditions in Asia and Oceania, including Australia, in maps as well, and thereby to achieve a comprehensive worldwide review of the known and ascertainable distribution of brucellosis, was not, however, practicable.) Information available from these parts of the world, especially from Asia, is so fragmentary that the great expense required for the compilation of the map did not seem justified. On the other hand it seemed desirable to collate and document these data which had been acquired as a basis for future research. It is to be hoped that, at a later date, when more comprehensive data become available, the Heidelberg Academy will be able to decide to support a cartographic presentation of the occurrence of brucellosis in these parts of the world as well.

Last, but not least, the intensive research carried out by bacteriologists had led to the discovery of new species of *Brucella*, such as *B. ovis, B. canis* and *B. neotomae*. Further types − such as Type 4 of *B. suis* which occurs in reindeer and caribou − were identified. Though these new species and types, which are undoubtedly to be classed with the *brucellae*, have achieved regional significance in places, the three classic species *B. melitensis, B. abortus* and *B. suis* remain epidemiologically and agriculturally the most important the world over.

Based on the data collected by the author in Europe, Africa and America, the new maps present the status up to 1976/77. In the compilation of the maps and the presentation of the situation in individual regions the author was aided by his own experience in his veterinary practice in Africa.

The maps are intended to stimulate fresh research into the distribution as well as the preconditions leading to more or less severe occurrence of brucellosis in different geographical regions. It is the only way to reduce the serious losses this disease causes among domestic animals and to protect human health. It is not without reason that brucellosis is internationally recognised, in the WHO and FAO alike, as one of the most significant animal diseases, causing chronic and insidious damage to animal stocks and thereby resulting in losses over the course of years and decades, the financial costs of which can only be estimated with difficulty. The encroachment upon human health too − assuming the age distribution follows the normal pattern − striking the active and working-age group especially, is not easy to assess because of the often chronic and not easily diagnosed form of the disease. Brucellosis is thus not only of economic importance for cattle breeding and food supplies, but also has a socio-medical significance that should not be lightly dismissed.

All those who have an interest in research into brucellosis and, by no means least, in the control of the disease are — together with the author — indebted to the governing body of the Heidelberg Academy of Sciences for making possible this work and assisting its progress throughout. This help has included travel grants which allowed the author to visit research centres concerned with brucellosis in Europe and overseas, as well making available the means for the printing of the multichrome maps. The compilation of the maps was made possible only thanks to the generous help of Professor Jusatz and his long experience in the cartographic presentation of disease patterns. His colleagues who carried out the cartographic work up to the stage of montage and printing by the „Kartographisches Atelier und Offsetdruckerei Henning Wocke" in Karlsruhe also deserve mention here. The Geomedical Research Unit and the Academy itself recognised the necessity of — and were immediately prepared to mount — a questionnaire survey addressed to the relevant authorities for the countries of all continents. The authorities and ministries of those countries which supported the author by responding to these enquiries, like those institutes he was able to visit, deserve especial thanks here. Thanks are also due to the Springer publishing house in Heidelberg who were engaged in production of this supplementary volume of the series. For the English translation my thanks go to Dr. Anthony Hellen of the Department of Geography, University of Newcastle upon Tyne, and Mrs Inge Hellen. With the publication of the maps and the supplementary volume the Geomedical Research Unit of the Heidelberg Academy of Sciences has once again fulfilled its purpose of continuing the description of diseases and updating their cartographic presentation, the distribution of which had once been known, to the latest state of knowledge.

Mannheim, March 1982   Wilhelm Wundt

Contents

Enclosures:
Map-Plate 1: Brucellosis. Distribution in Man, Domestic
and Wild Animals in Europe
Brucellose. Verbreitung beim Menschen, bei Haustieren
und beim Wild in Europa

Map-Plate 2: Brucellosis. Distribution in Man, Domestic
and Wild Animals in Africa

Map-Plate 3: Brucellosis. Distribution in Man, Domestic
and Wild Animals in The Americas

Back of Map 3:
Special Map 1: Brucellosis Incidence in Man in USA in
the Period 1968–1977. 10 year average of reported cases
per 100,000 inhabitants

1 Introduction

The term brucellosis is applied to a group of closely related infectious diseases, which are caused by germs of the bacterial species *Brucella*. They occur all over the world. Man almost always receives the infection from infected animals, whereas transmission from man to man usually does not occur. Measures against this anthropozoonosis will therefore always have to aim at the control and eradication of the disease in the animal reservoir as well. The damage done to the economy (abortions, infertility, loss of milk and meat in the case of domestic animals) and to the public health (through chronic infections and absenteeism from work among the populace) by this zoonosis amounts to millions of dollars in the countries affected by it. According to statements by the WHO (1975) about half a million fall ill from it every year.

The bases for meaningful and economic measures in the national as well as in the international context are surveys and proven data on incidence. Geomedical maps provide a synopsis of the state of knowledge on the extent of the disease at the particular time, and at the same time maps of brucellosis distribution show the great changes that have taken place in the countries concerned since the last cartographic overview by W. Wundt in 1961 as a result of increased surveys and thus increased knowledge and intensified measures which were adopted in those states.

1.1 Brucella Species and Biotypes

The germs are small, coccoide, gram-negative, rod-like bacteria of about $0.5\,\mu -1.5\,\mu$ in length and $0.5\,\mu -0.7\,\mu$ in breadth. They are not encapsulated, immobile and sporeless; they grow in a strictly aerobic atmosphere at an optimal temperature of $37\,°C$ (within the range of $20-40\,°C$) and an optimal pH of $6.6-7.4$.

Strains of the brucella species *B. abortus* and *B. ovis* mostly require a supplementary CO_2 atmosphere of $5-10\%$ for their initial isolation. Brucellae are parasites of mammals with a wide spectrum of hosts and a facultive intracellular reproduction. They are extremely well adapted to the interior milieu of their host organisms. Their isolation and differentiation therefore requires special media and the existence of well-equipped laboratories and staff well trained in handling infectious material (laboratory infections!) — a fact which ought not to be forgotten when seeking and evaluating geomedically utilizeable investigation data.

Table 1. Characters differentiating the species and biotypes in the genus Brucella

Species and Biotypes		Reference neo-type strain[2]	CO₂ Req.	H₂S Prod.	Growth on dye media[3]			Agglutin. with[4]			Lysis by phage at RTD[1]				Substrates metabolized oxidatively										
					B.F. b)	Th. a)	Th. b)	A	M	R	Tb	Wb	Bk	R	L-alanine	L-asparagine	L-glutamic acid	L-arabinose	D-galactose	D-ribose	D-glucose	i-erythritol	D-xylose	L-arginine	L-lysine
B. melitensis	1	16 M	–	–	+	–	+	–	+	–	–	–	+	–	+	+	+	–	–	–	+	+	–	–	–
	2	62/9	–	–	+	–	+	+	+	–	Biotyp 1 – 3				Biotyp 1 – 3										
	3	Ether	–	+	+	–	+	+	+	–																
B. abortus	1	544	+(–)	+	–	–	–	+	–	–	+	+	+	+ R only	+	+	+	+	+	+	+	+	–	–	–
	2	86/8/59	+(–)	+	–	–	–	+	–	–	Biotyp 1 – 9				Biotyp 1 – 9										
	3	Tulya	+(–)	+	+	+	+	+	–	–																
	4	292	+(–)	+	+	–	–	–	+	–																
	5	B 3196	+(–)	–	+	–	+	–	+	–																
	6	870	–	–	+	–	+	+	+	–																
	7	63/75	–	–(+)	+	–	+	+	+	–																
	8	N.A.	+	–	+	–	+	–	+	–																
	9	C 68	–	+	+	–	+	–	+	–																
B. suis	1	1330	–	+	–	+	–	+	–	–	+	+			–	–	–	+	+	+	+	+	+	+	+
	2	Thomsen	–	–	–	–	–	+	–	–	Biotyp 1 – 4				–	–	+	+	+	+	+	+	+	–	–
	3	686	–	–	+	+	–	+	–	–					–	–	+	–	–	+	+	+	+	+	+
	4	40	–	–	+	–	+	–	+	–					–	–	+	–	–	–	+	+	+	+	+
B. neotomae	5	K 33	–	+	–	–	+	+	–	–	±	+	+		+	+	+	+	+	±	+	+	+	–	–
B. ovis		63/290	+	–	+	+	+	–	–	+	–	–			+	+	+	–	–	–	–	–	–	–	–
B. canis		R M 6/66	–	–	–	–	+	–	–	+	–	–			–	–	+	–	+	+	+	±	–	+	+

1 RTD=Routine Test Dilution; +=QO₂N values ≥ 50; –=QO₂N values ≤ 50; Tb=Tbilisi phage; Bk=Berkeley phage; R=Antirough phage; DL-citrulline and ornithine give the same reactions as L-arginine Wb=Weybridge phage;
2 Reference strains or biotypes available from National Type Culture Collection, Colindale, England or from the American Type Culture Collection, Rockville, Md, USA
3 Certified dyes (National Aniline Division, Allied Chemical & Dye Co., New York) at concentrations of: a) 1/25 000; b) 1/50 000; B.F.=Basic Fuchsin; Th=Thionine

Table 2. Main host reservoirs of *Brucella* species and biotypes

Species	Biotypes	Main Hosts	Side Hosts	Pathogenic to Man
B. melitensis	1 – 3	goat, sheep	cattle	+
B. abortus	1 – 9	cattle, buffalo	horse	+
B. suis	1	pig	cattle	+
	2	pig, hare	cattle	+
	3	pig	cattle	+
	4	reindeer	?	+
B. ovis	1	sheep	?	?
B. canis	1	dog	?	+
B. neotomae	1	desert wood rat (Neotoma lepida, Thomas)	?	?

Source: Joint FAO/WHO Expert Committee on Brucellosis (1971) W. Wundt (1956)

Taxonomically the *genus Brucella* comprises 6 species, which differ in their host specificity, epidemiology, pathogenicity to man and animals and in their metabolic behaviour (see Tables 1 and 2). The species can be distinguished by their oxidative utilization of certain amino acids and carbohydrates as well as by their sensitivity to bacteriophages, whereas the Brucella species *B. melitensis*, *B. abortus* and *B. suis* can be divided into different biotypes[1] with the aid of the analysis of their CO_2 requirements, their H_2S production, their growth on cultural media containing dyestuffs, and their reaction to monospecific antisera. This resulted in an excellent tool for the discovery and clarification of epidemiological linkages. Unfortunately in the countries affected by it isolation and typification of brucellae is not yet carried out to such an extent as would appear to be worthwhile for geomedical evaluation of the existing data.

The brucella species are specialized on certain main and side hosts.

B. melitensis is the germ causing the Undulating or Malta fever in man. Its preferred main reservoir hosts are goats, sheep and wild ruminants (e.g. antelopes). Side hosts are the animals of their immediate environs, such as cattle and the carnivores – dog, jackal and hyena.

B. abortus, the germ causing Bang's disease in man and contagious abortions in bovines, uses domestic cattle and water buffalo as its main reservoir hosts, and in endemic areas sheep, goats, pigs, dogs, foxes, jackals and hyenas as side hosts.

B. suis prefers the domestic pig as its main reservoir host and in Africa as side host the goat, in Europe *B. suis biotype 2* also prefers the hare.

B. suis, biotype 4 has only been found in man and in the domesticated and the wild reindeer or caribou (*Rangifer tarandus granti, L* and *R. tarandi groenlandicus, L*) as well as in the carnivores wolf, dog and fox feeding on it.

---

1 The term "biotype" was retained because the classification of *brucellae* within the taxon "species" is based on biochemical as well as serological criteria and, furthermore, because the reader – where he happens not to be a microbiologist – will tend to be more familiar with this expression than with "biovar", "serovar" or other terms which have now been introduced into the nomenclature of microbiology.

B. canis having been discovered in beagle dogs in the U.S.A. by Carmichael as late as 1968 has been established as a distinct species of Brucella by now, as the germ of contagious abortion among cannel dogs as well as stray dogs in other countries. Isolated cases have even occurred among humans, mainly laboratory workers.

B. ovis finds its chief reservoir hosts only in sheep; side hosts are unknown. In the ram this species causes infectious epididymitis with frequent infertility, in ewes it leads to abortions. Again, some isolated cases have been reported in man.

B. neotomae appears to be confined to the American desert wood rat (*Neotoma lepida Thomas*). Nothing is known about infections in man.

1.2 The Chain of Natural Infection Cycles

All these brucella species pass through complete cycles of infection in the host animal species of their preference. But, since they are polycyclic with the exception of *B. canis, B. ovis* and *B. neotomae,* they do transfer to other animal species and also with ease to man, if the ecological-epizootic conditions are favourable.

Within the epidemiology of the disease, however, man has to be regarded as an epidemiological "cul de sac" of the disease. Man acquires it almost exclusively from infected domestic animals, and – as a hunter in Africa and America – evidently directly from game, such as antelopes and wild boars, as well. Transmissions from man to man are rare, and play practically no role in the epidemiology of the disease. Human brucellosis is therefore to be regarded as an anthropozoonosis, and can only be considered in close connection with the actual brucellosis situation among domestic and wild animals.

The natural cycles of infection from animal to animal and from animal to man are shown in Fig. 1.

Different species of brucella, though preferring specific main hosts, are not strongly host-specific, as indicated by the direction of the arrows in Fig. 1. Apart from the domestic animals mentioned above, such as cattle, sheep, goat, pig and dog, others like the horse, donkey, greater and lesser camel (alpacas) and the hare must be included as natural reservoirs of the agents for man.

Fig. 1 presents a general chain of infection, the members of which are populated by various host animal – and brucella species. The size of the circles indicates not only the epidemiological and economic significance of the animal brucellosis under consideration for man, but also the epizootiological significance of the individual animal groups for each other, as large and small ruminants, pigs, reindeer and infected carnivores.

This group of domestic animal brucellosis is intersected – as if by a short-circuiting chain of infection – by the range of cycles of wild animals, especially by the wild ungulates (like buffalo, gazelle and zebra, which form part of the animal collective) and wild carnivores, which are partly separated from, but partly connected with the domestic animal cycles (indicated here as arrows pointing in opposite directions). Added to these are the brucellosis of poultry, particularly of waterfowls, and of wild rodents, especially rats and mice, and

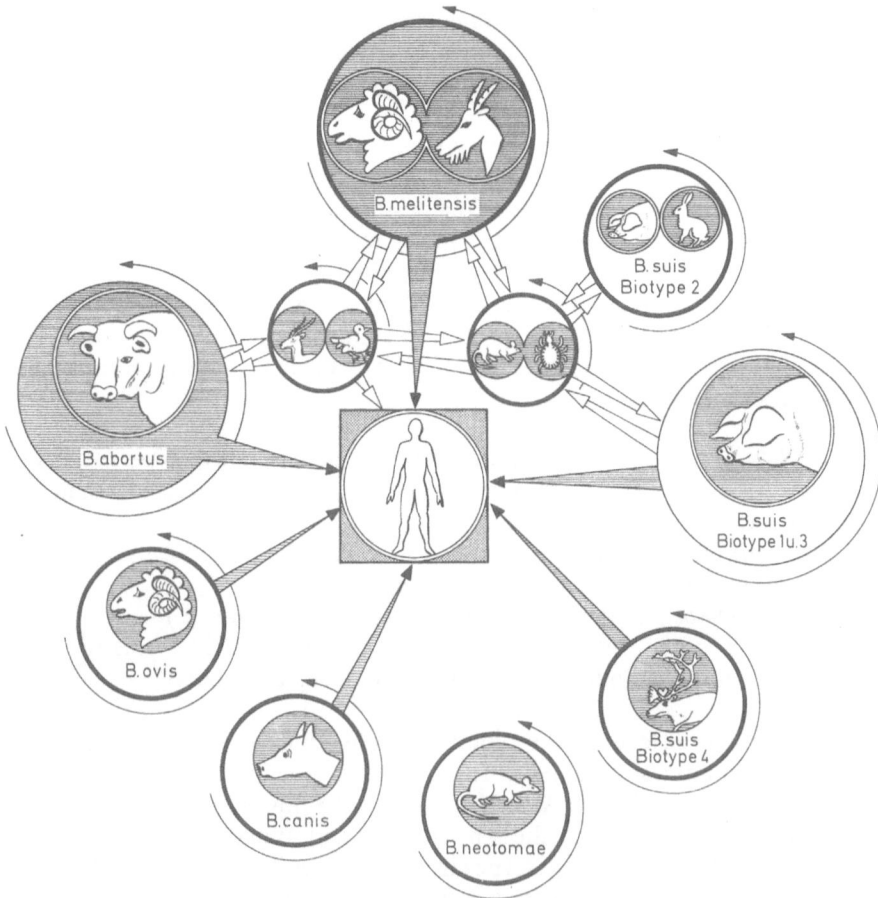

Fig. 1. Natural infection cycles of various brucella species

as potential vectors the blood-sucking arthropods like ticks, mites, midges and blood-sucking flies. But at present no unequivocal statements can be made on these (Remenzowa 1966).

Thus a quasi-threedimensional impression of a network of the disease epidemiology is created, the nodal points of which present individual units of the total process of brucellosis, which can only be correctly analyzed and evaluated in connection with the knowledge of the local epidemiological conditions. This broad spectrum of hosts makes it uncommonly difficult to take control measures against brucellosis.

1.3 Natural Foci in Wild Animals

Without detailed investigations there is thus no way of a priori determining which of the following four types of infection within the biozoonotic framework the natural foci determined in wild animals are part of.

1.3.1 Natural foci derived from domestic animals. Deviating from the normal behaviour of closed infection cycles brucellosis in wild animals appears to depend much on the presence of brucellosis foci in the domestic stock. It disappears as soon as the latter are eradicated.

The connecting link is probably supplied by aborted foetusses and foetal membranes, which, dragged around by carnivores are also capable of spreading the disease to hitherto brucellosis-free pastures and domestic herds.

Herbivores can also be infected orally and aerogenically via dust contaminated by *brucellae*. This occurs when germs are massively excreted during abortions and for weeks afterwards by domestic and wild animals alike in the lochial fluids, where they are protected against desiccation (e.g. infection of foxes by aborted pig foetusses, or of wolves through consumption of infected reindeer meat).

1.3.2 Natural foci also derived from domestic animals, but then persisting in wild animals for a long time and independently of domestic infected animals. The following examples can be quoted:
B. melitensis in the Saiga-antelope (*Saiga tatarica, L.*)
B. abortus in the bison (*Bison bison, L.*) or
B. abortus biotype 3 in the African buffalo (*Synceros caffer, L.*)

They are largely infections or re-infections of the wild forms of domesticated stock of the main reservoir hosts-cattle, sheep and goats.

1.3.3 The natural focus that originates in wild animals, but has so far not been found in the domestic animals. This concerns rodents, herbivores, and carnivores in the U.S.A., Africa, Australia and the U.S.S.R. Examples are:
B. neotomae, isolated from the American Desert Wood Rat (*Neotoma lepida, Thomas*), unclassified *brucella* types in *Rattus assimilis, Melomys* and *M. lutillus* in Queensland, Australia, *B. suis biotype 3* in *Arvicanthus niloticus* and *Mastomys natalensis* in Kenya and unstable biotypes in *Mus musculus* (FAO 1971).

1.3.4 Natural focus that originates in wild animals, but may also act as a source of infection for domestic animals. Here *B. suis biotype 2* may serve as an example, which has been established in the Europaean field hare (*Lepus europaeus, L.*) in Denmark as the original host, but can easily be transmitted to domestic pigs.

According to Pawlowski and Galuso (cit. Remenzowa, 1966) there may be natural foci of brucellosis consisting of different animal species, especially rats and ticks, which are parts in the chain of infection in the forest- and steppe-biocoenosis. Karkadinowkdaja (1936, 1937; cit. Remenzowa 1966) identified 11.8% (4/34) of the wild rats caught (*Rattus norwegicus, L.*) in the U.S.S.R and Bouatra (1970) 16.7% (2/12) in Morocco as being infected with brucellosis. Transmission takes place through the urin of rats and of other locally numerous rodents (ground squirrel, field mice and others).

Experiments have shown that brucellae multiply in ticks and remain alive in them for over 2 years (Remenzowa 1966). They are transmitted transovarially to the next generation of ticks without any loss of virulence. Nevertheless this route of transmission appears to be of little importance in the epizootiology of the disease compared with the three main routes of infection – peroral, aerogen and intrauterine – for mammals. Remenzowa (1951 cit. Parnas 1966), in the course of examining 11,267 ticks, which had been collected from brucellosis-infected animals, found only 7 (0.06%) infected with brucellae. Moreover it would be quite difficult to infect wild animals via this route, as the bacteraemic period in the mammal, where ticks could infect themselves is quite short and the natural resistance of wild animals is rather high so that this route of transmission may have only a little chance of success.

1.4 Permanent Carriers and Survival of the Germs

Brucellosis-infected animals need not show any disease symptoms yet may still present a continuous danger of infection for man in their capacity as chronic carriers and excreters of Brucellae (by way of infected milk, urine, faeces and in particularly large quantities in the foetal membranes, with the placenta and lochial excreta after abortion). Their considerable power of resistance, together with their ability to survive for long periods in liquids, animal products, for example milk, urine and manure, and in humid organic matter contribute to this,

e.g.	in tap water	at 18–21 °C	up to 60 days
	in dust	at 18–21 °C	42– 72 days
	in cattle manure, dry	at 18–21 °C	120–160 days
	in goats cheese	at 4– 8 °C	up to 180 days

(FAO 1971, Parnas et al. 1966, Weber 1980)

1.5 The Epidemiology of Human Brucellosis

As a zoonosis brucellosis is primarily an animal disease. Man becomes infected as a result of handling infected domestic animals, and the objects and products contaminated by them, and in some rare cases even when hunting – as for example by the primary source of infected game. The main sources of infection for man are therefore his domestic animals, like cattle, sheep, goats, pig and dog, but also the camel, alpaca, water buffalo, yak and domesticated reindeer in certain areas of the world (see Fig. 1). Transmission from man to man practically never takes place.

1.5.1 Routes of Infection

a) Per Contact. Man can become infected by way of minute wounds on the skin or in the mucous membrane of the mouth, but also conjunctivally when assisting at animal birth or abortion, or even when preparing or manufacturing animal products (such as milk, cheese, butter, cream, meat, wool).

b) Peroral. The second most important route of infection is via the digestive system; after the peroral intake of germs together with raw, *brucellae*-infected milk or products made from it (e.g. fresh sheep or goat cheese in the Mediterranean region). Even consumption of insufficiently cooked meat from cattle, sheep, goat, pig or game are potential sources of danger (e.g. goat meat in East Africa, raw reindeer meat among Eskimos). Another possibility of infection is the consumption of raw vegetables and salads which have become contaminated by the manure or urine of infected animals ("Top dressing").

c) Aerogenically by Inhalation of Aerosols or Dust. By inhaling *brucellae*-containing dust (in stables, on routes of travel on the hoof, drove routes, pastures, animal transport vehicles) ostic or vaccine laboratories. Particularly at risk are the occupational groups who find themselves in constant close contact with animals and their products by the nature of their profession such as butchers and workers in slaughterhouses and deep-freezing plants, wool washers, tanners, farmers, veterinarians and laboratory staff.

1.5.2 Epidemiological Patterns. However, the probability of becoming infected with brucellosis in a country depends on a definite epidemiological pattern of factors:

a) the degree of spread in the animal reservoir,
b) the species of animals that are kept,
c) the methods and forms of animal husbandry,
d) the size of the herds,
e) the customs and practices of people in their handling of animals, as well as of the production, preparation and consumption of food,
f) the standard of personal and environmental hygiene,
g) the local and seasonal climatic conditions and their consequences (e.g. on the personal hygiene and the intensity of contact with animals) (lack of water in periods of drought or cold, crowding factor, etc.).

The combination of these diverse factors and their variable evaluation are decisive for the multiplicity of the local epidemiological situation and disease pattern, and at the same time the background to the difficulty of any successful anti-brucellosis campaign. It also implies that regional geomedical presentations of the disease constantly require re-examinations of their local validity through separate local investigations.

1.6 The Disease Manifestation in Man

The course the disease takes in man depends on the infecting *brucella* species, the dosage and virulence of the germ, the general condition of resistance and immunity of the patient and the frequency, duration and intensity of the contact. The *incubation period* varies greatly, between 1 and 3 weeks, and in some cases even up to 6 to 7 months.

Brucella melitensis and *B. suis* infections tend to be more severe than those caused by *B. abortus.*

Three forms of the disease, with more or less flowing transitions, can be distinguished:

1. *Non-apparent infection* with a tendency to a complete cure without persistence of germs. The contact with brucellae is serologically provable.
2. *Acute and sub-acute brucellosis* with generalisation and cure without persistence of germs. A reinfection is possible. The disease is characterized by weakness, fever, lassitude, bouts of shivering and sweating, pain in the body, joints, muscles and especially in the head, and loss of weight (in this order of frequencies).
3. *Chronic brucellosis,* which many patients reach immediately after the non-apparent infection or after passing through the sub-acute phase. Patients with diminished resistance or frequent and persistent contact with brucellosis are particularly at risk. There is no tendency to cure.

After the generalisation the brucellae colonize especially in the bones, joints, nerves and brain, vessels and in the heart and sexual organs, with corresponding symptoms and consequences. Probably as a result of endotoxin and septic shock caused by the gramnegative brucellae, foetal death and abortion may occur in pregnant women (Schreyer et al. 1980).

Attacks of mostly intermittent or constant fever, together with its concomitant symptoms and a great reduction in working efficiency are a striking feature.

Evidence of the germ, though difficult, is the only proof (from blood or the spinal cord). A large palette of serological test methods enables the investigator to make a diagnosis of suspected brucellosis.

These three forms of the disease with their objective and/or subjective symptoms are distinct from that of the *hyper-ergic status* which is attained by many patients after their recovery from brucellosis. They feel fine and free from symptoms, there is no further evidence of germs, but serological tests continue to show positive or at least suspected results, which are, however, to be judged only as proof of an earlier antigen contact (Vanek 1976).

The masking of brucellosis in a variety of disease patterns makes it difficult for the clinician not to mistake it for another disease. There may be untold human suffering if brucellosis as the real cause of the disease is not detected for years, and the chronic damage which has resulted remains untreated. Case histories of up to 25 years' duration have been observed (Spink 1975).

1.7 The Course of the Disease Among Animals

Brucellosis is above all a disease of the herd. If an animal of a herd is infected the entire band must be suspected of having contracted brucellosis. The courses taken by the disease in cattle, sheep, goats, pigs and dogs agree in their essential points.

After the disease's introduction (usually by buying-in of an infected animal) the first infection tends to pass unnoticed. Contrary to the process in man, the colonization of brucellae in the reproductive organs constitutes the main event during the chronic stage, which is accompanied – according to species – by the more or less vigorous production of erythritol. This has the effect of promoting growth in the brucellae. Female animals, having developed an endometritis with a necrosis of the placenta, experience the death of the foetus and abortion. Occasional abortions are scarcely noticed. Usually only the so-called "abortion storm" causes alarm, when epidemic miscarriages among cattle, sheep, goats etc. affect up to 25 per cent of a herd. Abortions are frequently accompanied by premature or stillbirths among other animals of the herd. Sheep and goats tend to give birth to weak lambs and kids. Because these require more intensive care and "mothering" by man they constitute a particular risk of infection to him.

Together with the discharged placenta, the foetal membranes and lochial secretions the aborting animals continue to pass masses of brucellae in the course of the following days and weeks. Thus a rapid dispersion of the disease and the maintenance of a chain of infection among man and animals are ensured (see Fig. 1).

Abortion among cattle, sheep and goats is often followed by the colonization of brucellae in the udder, resulting in years of excreting brucellae with the milk and the corresponding risks of infection for man (WHO 1971). Milk production declines. At the same times there is a tendency to infertility, caused by endometritides in the female and orchitides and epididymitides in the male animals. In some cases the joints have been affected by bursitis and tendovaginitis, especially in Sanga Zebu cattle infected by *B. abortus, biotype 3* in Africa.

1.8 The Significance of Brucellosis for Public Health and for the Economy

There are three reasons for the continuing worldwide importance of brucellosis:

1. It is a highly relevant health problem for man in the affected areas.
2. It causes annually serious losses in the livestock industry of the economy.
3. It is difficult to diagnose in man.

Measures against it in the animal reservoir prove to be expensive and protracted.

In affected areas chiefly engaged in cattle keeping, and where the consumption of untreated cow's milk and milk products is common, *B. abortus* is frequent. This does not, however, attract much attention since the progress of the infections is rather protracted. Infections with *B. melitensis* and *B. suis* in areas engaged predominantly in the rearing of sheep, goats and pigs lead to serious cases of the disease and to complications in man. Thousands of fresh cases of brucellosis are reported from these areas (Italy, Spain, Greece) every year (WHO 1979). The losses of manpower and income as a result of physical and psychic reduction in efficiency are difficult to assess, however. The entire damage annually inflicted upon the economy by brucellosis in the animal herds is considerable. The direct loss of meat (as a result of abortions, infertility and weight losses) in infected herds of cattle was estimated to be 15 per cent, and in the case of milk (falling off in milk production) at 20 per cent per infected cow (U.S. Dept. of Agriculture 1972). In 1957, before measures against brucellosis had begun to be applied, these losses amounted to a total value of US $ 66 million in the German Federal Republic, to US $ 81.6 million in France foether in 1960 (WHO 1962), and in Latin America and the U.S.A. combined to about US $ 700 million per year (Abdussalam 1976). Losses in the flocks of sheep and goats are hardly less, relatively speaking. A complete elimination of brucellosis would accordingly result in high annual gains.

Freedom from brucellosis is defined as an annual infection rate of less than 0.001 per cent of the animals (Schreiber 1974).

The costs of measures against brucellosis are by no means small. In the Federal Republic of Germany the annual expenditure on measures against both bovine brucellosis and tuberculosis together amounted to US $ 50 million (WHO 1962).

Wherever it is attempted it proves to be a protracted business, extending over several years and requiring practicable legislative measures, a well informed and highly motivated public (especially among the farming community), well-trained doctors, veterinary surgeons and laboratory staff, financial and laboratory-technical provisions, as well as good, flexible planning, organisation and co-operation.

This explains why completed programmes of control and eradication have so far been reported only by industrialized states which are not only financially strong, but are also supported by the necessary high level of agricultural and hygiene development.

The creeping and chronically damaging character of brucellosis on the other hand explains why, in the developing countries, the true significance of brucellosis for the nation's health as well as for the nation's economy is still largely unrecognized or at least not taken note of in the face of the other acute epidemic diseases. Measures against brucellosis can hardly be expected to receive priority there, although it would be most helpful to those who require a high intake of protein in view of the high annual birthrate, and the need to develop their vital agriculture as fast as possible. The direct gains attainable by eliminating brucellosis would exceed everything in the areas presently affected that can be achieved through annual rates of increased output in animal husbandry.

Since the expense required to reach this aim is correspondingly high, and the success of measures against brucellosis depends upon recognition of the true extent of the problem – together with well co-ordinated efforts carried out on different levels at the same time – for many countries this aim inevitably remains one in the distant future.

The statement by the WHO Expert Committee on Brucellosis is therefore to be endorsed without reservation.

"Brucellosis has proved to be one of the most difficult problems of disease" and "in many countries of the world it contributes to the low standard of living in the most far-reaching way" (WHO 1964).

The mapping of the present epidemiological situation of the disease is therefore intended to actively support this process of recognition and successful campaigning against brucellosis.

2 The Mapping of the Occurrence of Brucellosis in Man and in Domestic and Wild Animals

The mapping of a disease like brucellosis, which depends upon a variety of factors and occurs in man and animals alike, poses special problems for the medical cartographer.

Not only does the broad spectrum of germs and hosts need to be displayed, but the worldwide development of animal husbandry, the mass keeping of animals and animal transports, in connection with widely differing successes in the diagnosis and control of the disease, dynamically contribute to the fluctuations in the epidemiological picture.

At the same time it is now no longer possible to make statements on the routes of importation and the spread of the disease from one country to another, since the international ties of dealing in livestock and animal products have become so close and interwoven.

The distribution picture of brucellosis has undergone great changes as a result of national control programmes including regular or sporadic monitoring of its spread in many countries since the seventies. It therefore seems to be advisible to portray the *status quo* by publishing a few new maps as visual aids, and to map afresh the distribution of brucellosis which was first shown by Wundt (1961) in the *World Atlas of Epidemic Diseases* twenty years ago.

2.1 Material and Methods

The methodology of data collection, and especially the evaluation of data from so-called "grey" (i.e. non-computerized) literature, such as annual and laboratory reports of departments of human and veterinary medicine has been referred to in detail in another place (Thimm and Wundt 1976). Particularly useful for this — apart from individual investigation of reference collections — were the data pool available in the Animal Health Yearbook of the FAO in Rome for the period 1968–1974, the bulletins of the OIE in Paris, the bulletins and statistical reports of the WHO in Geneva, the Boletin de la Oficina Sanitaria Panamericana of the WHO in Washington ánd the computer search in the Medlars System of the DIMDI, Cologne. Last, but not least, the libraries of the FAO in Rome and the WHO in Buenos Aires, of the World Brucellosis Reference Laboratory, Weybridge, England, of the Tropical Institute of the Faculty of Veterinary Medicine at Maison Alfort, Paris, and the Institute for Comparative Tropical Medicine in Munich proved a veritable treasure trove of rare reports on the occurrence and frequency of brucellosis in individual countries. Another way to collect information was with the aid of questionnaires which were sent by the Geomedical Research Unit of the Heidelberg Academy of Sciences to the Departments of Human and Veterinary Medicine of all countries.

The questionnaires enquired into the self-assessment of the countries in respect of the position of brucellosis from the public health and economic points of view. The response rate amounted to 40 of the 150 countries which had been approached.

2.2 Mapping of the Occurrence

In presenting the occurrence of brucellosis preference was given to those cases which were bacteriologically established, but in most cases it was necessary to make do with serological results.

Above all the maps were intended to represent the evidence of brucellosis frequencies in man. In order to plot the animal reservoir which positively forms a constituent part of the understanding of human brucellosis, the brucella species which had been isolated in animals were put in different colours and areal forms below the relevant animal symbols, and the reported frequency of occurrence indicated in special hachures. The figure indicated here should always be regarded as a minimum number of cases, with the dark figure varying from country to country.

2.3 Mapping of Frequency (Prevalence, Incidence)

The maps were intended to show the *prevalence*, which is nothing but an inventory at a specific moment in the disease frequency of a certain species population, or the *incidence*, which introduces the concept of a period into the inventory of a specific moment, a quasi-presentation of a film sequence of a dynamic infection and recovery process over a period under observation. Frequently only case data or prevalence data of sample surveys were available, for the setting up of an official enquiry into incidence requires every country to have a laboratory- and communication system in the human and veterinary medicine sector which functions well. Where both the indices were available, for example the number of reported human cases of brucellosis per 100,000 inhabitants per annum and the number of patients infected in one outbreak of the disease, the incidence was always preferred (see Table 3 Incidence Reading Key).

Difficulties in the selection of indices for mapping arose with the information on infection rates from veterinary medicine. Here the sample, i.e. survey results, must unequivocally be preferred to those on prevalence if no incidence rates covering several years are obtainable from national offices concerned with animal health.

2.4 The Herd as an Epizootiological Entity

Brucellosis researchers have long been aware that the real epizootiological entity is not an animal population scattered over an entire area, but an *animal herd,* whereas man as the real contact with the animal reservoir must always also be evaluated as an individual single case. However, in areas where the common grazing of herds is practiced, the area or village are more of an epizootiological entity than the separate herds. In consequence the epizootiological point of view demands that quite different examination and evelution criteria be deployed for this disease.

In the case of brucellosis in man the incidence of individual cases per 100,000 inhabitants per annum, preferably as a mean value for a five year period, is primarily to be referred to, whereas among animals the epizootiological unit of a herd is to be used to the same extent as the rate of infection for individual animals. Thus it has therefore become a tendency in recent years, especially at the FAO Centre for Animal Health, which specializes in these matters, to apply a combined incidence-evaluation key for individual animals and herds. This has only the one disadvantage of integrating too great a number of groups, thus offering cartography too few distinctions for display of the local occurrence of the disease (FAO 1974).

2.5 Key for Evaluation

We have therefore arranged for a further sub-division of this key, and the enclosed maps are compiled on that basis (see Table 3 of Reading Key, Thimm and Nauwerck 1974).

Table 3. Combined incidence reading key on an individual and herd base

Individual incidence %	Herd incidence %	Reading of the incidence
f	f	free
0 – 5.9	0 – 10.9	sporadic
6.0 – 15.9	11.0 – 20.9	low
16.0 – 25.0	21.0 – 30.0	moderate
above 25.0	above 30.0	high
?	?	suspected but not confirmed

2.6 The Mapping of Further Information on Epidemiological Details

Besides official data there is the possibility of making use of some reports at regional and district level, in particular of those on state legislative and control measures, which permit conclusions to be drawn in respect of the occurrence and frequency of the disease. To manage without them would mean to confine oneself to statistically guaranteed surveys of official case data enquiries. Epidemiologically, however, it would create a rather fragmentary picture. Entire areas, as for example the African continent or Eastern Asia, could not even be presented according to their disease epidemiology if they were based on these exact mathematical criteria alone. But the very search for and evaluation of

Table 4. Incidence and special hints to epidemiology

Sign	Legend
f	Country is free of disease from the beginning or after disease control
−	Not recorded; obviously not present
(−)	Not recorded; probably not present
?	Suspected but not confirmed
+!	Disease only recently recognised in country
(+)	Exceptional occurrence
+..	Disease exists; distribution and incidence entirely unknown
+∅	Confined to certain regions
+	Low incidence
++	Sporadic incidence
+++	Moderate incidence
++++	High incidence
+/	Disease much reduced, but still exists
...	No information available

Source: FAO Animal Health Year Book 1974, modified

reports and publications of these "grey areas" of papers, which are frequently not included in the annual reports of the Department of Human and Veterinary Medicine embraced by the Medlars System, also holds the fascination and the task of geomedical cartography. It is a task because only the first "special" contributions mentioning occurrence, frequency and characteristics of the disease in those countries retrospectively achieve the accumulation of energies which lead on to the actual control of the disease and exact reporting, and may finally end with success in the elimination of the disease (see Table 4).

With this approach medical cartography is able to put out a range of measuring feelers which are capable of registering the dynamics of a disease's progress over a long period, and thus to indicate *trends*.

3 Results of the Mapping of Brucellosis Occurrence

3.1 Brucellosis Occurrence in Europe and in the Mediterranean Countries

As a result of at times decades of successful measures of control against brucellosis the European continent no longer constitutes a uniform region of brucellosis distribution.

3.1.1 Animal Reservoirs. In the cooler and wetter countries of northern, western, central and eastern Europe, cattle — apart from pigs — are the main producers of meat and milk of animal origin, whereas the goat predominates in southern Europe. This may be explained by the plant-ecological features of a sclerophyllous vegetation around the Mediterranean Sea which permits the intensive breeding of goats.

Accordingly *B. abortus,* the agent of Bang's disease in man, which finds its main animal reservoir in cattle, frequently occurs in the former areas, whereas *B. melitensis,* the agent of Malta fever, is found more often in southern Europe and those countries which border the Mediterranean Sea, as well as in the Asian areas of the Soviet Union.

After the elimination of *B. abortus* from most countries in Europe the latent problem of *B. suis* among pigs, however, remains. As in the U.S.A., the brucellosis infections concentrate increasingly on slaughterhouse workers, caused primarily by *B. suis* and secondarily by *B. abortus.*

3.1.2 Frequency of Occurrence and Distribution of Brucellosis in Man and Animals (Table 5). Depending on the animal reservoir and the local conditions of climate and animal husbandry, as well as of the energy and efficiency of the control measures taken, five sub-regions or zones of frequency of disease distribution can be distinguished: they range from the brucellosis-free status in countries in the north of Europe to areas of high grade endemic infection in some parts of the Mediterranean region. On the whole, however, a spatial trend showing considerable decrease from South to North can be observed in almost all countries together with a declining trend over time, compared with the last mapping undertaken by W. Wundt (1961) in the *World Atlas of Epidemic Diseases.*

3.1.2.1 Zone I: Brucellosis-Free Zone. This zone is situated exclusively in northern Europe. The map particularly emphasises that the Scandinavian countries in northern Europe have in parts been free from brucellosis for more than twenty years – Norway since 1952, Sweden since 1957, Finland since 1960, Denmark since 1962. Iceland and the Channel Islands are likewise free from brucellosis.

The smaller the number of animal reservoirs and the rate of incidence per individual animal or animal herd, the easier it is for a country to rid itself of brucellosis. At least in parts, this explains the present freedom of those countries from brucellosis. From the very beginning they suffered only from bovine brucellosis. *B. melitensis* and *B. ovis* never arose in those countries, and *B. suis* neither in Finland nor in Norway. In Sweden the last case in a pig was registered in 1957. Denmark still reports occasional cases of *B. suis* in pigs.

3.1.2.2 Zone II: With Sporadic Brucellosis Occurrence.

Large areas in the entire European area have already almost reached the goal of becoming brucellosis-free.

Thus only sporadic occurrences (0–0.59 cases per 100,000 inhabitants per year) are reported in western and central Europe, including the Netherlands, Belgium, the German Federal Republic, Austria and Switzerland, Poland, Czechoslovakia, Roumania and Bulgaria, and in the southern European countries of Yugoslavia and Turkey.

Bovine Brucellosis in Zone II. Switzerland, Czechoslovakia, Roumania and Bulgaria are already free from bovine brucellosis.

Occurrence in the Netherlands, Luxembourg, the German Federal Republic and Austria are the exception; they are sporadic in Belgium, of a low grade frequency in Poland and Yugoslavia, and of a medium one in Turkey.

Brucellosis Among Sheep and Goats in Zone II. In the Federal Republic of Germany *B. melitensis* brucellosis among sheep and goats only counts as a sporadically recurring problem, due to the migration of flocks which graze in the warmer areas of Alsace-Lorraine/France in winter and return to the south German pastures in the spring, sporadically infected with brucellosis.

Poland, Czechoslovakia, Roumania and Bulgaria, the four east European countries of endemic grade II, are free from *B. melitensis* brucellosis, according to their own reports.

B. melitensis brucellosis continues to be a problem among goats in Yugoslavia and Turkey, these countries bordering on the Mediterranean Sea, and among sheep in Turkey, but both cases are regarded as belonging to the "low grade" category. However, the reports on human cases do not reveal how these affect man. Yugoslavia has been free from ovine brucellosis caused by *B. melitensis* since 1972. In Roumania, Yugoslavia and Turkey *B. ovis* was found in sheep (see Map Brucellosis Incidence in Europe).

Swine Brucellosis in Zone II. Swine brucellosis, caused by *B. suis,* presents quite a different picture in this endemic zone II. The occurrence in Belgium, Luxembourg, Austria, Switzerland, Poland and Czechoslovakia is classified as sporadic, whereas it remains a low grade problem in the Federal Republic of Germany, due in part at least to cross-infections with *B. suis biotype 2* from the field hare, and a medium to high grade problem in the pig herds of Yugoslavia and Roumania.

Wild animal reservoirs of *B. suis biotype 2* in hares (*Lepus europaeus,* L) have been reported from the German Federal Republic, Austria, Poland, Czechoslovakia, the German Democratic Republic and Yugoslavia (FAO 1974).

Table 5. Brucellosis incidence in Europe (Period 1968 – 1975)

Country	Reported human cases per 100,000 P.p.a.	Cattle B. abortus	Sheep B. abortus	Sheep B. mel.	Sheep B. ovis	Goat B. mel.	Swine B. suis	Game and other domestic animals
Zone I (declared brucellosis free)		free since						
Norway	–	1952	–	–	–	–	–	–
Sweden	0.04	1957	–	–	–	–	since 1957	–
Finland	–	1961	–	–	–	–	–	–
Denmark	–	1962	–	–	–	–	(+)	(+) Hare
Iceland	–	always	–	–	–	–	–	–
Channel Islands	–	always	–	–	–	–	–	–
Zone II (Sporadic Incidence, 0 – 0.59 cases / 100,000 Pop. p.a.)								
Netherlands	0.05	(+)	–	–	–	–	–	–
Belgium	0.06	+	–	–	–	–	(+)	–
Luxembourg	0.53	(+)	+	+	–	–	(+)	–
Fed. Rep. Germany	0.13	(+)	+	+	–	–	+	(+) Hare
Austria	0.56	(+)	(–)	–	–	–	(+)	(+) Hare
Switzerland	0.27	– 1963	–	–	+/	–	+	(+) Hare
Germ. Dem. Rep.	0.59	+	+	–	–	–	+	+Ø Hare
Poland	0.56+	++/	–	–	–	–	(+)	+ Hare
CSSR	0.01	– 1964	–	–	++	–	(+)	(+)
Roumania	0.06+	– 1969	–	–	+	–	++	
Bulgaria	0.11	– 1958	–	– 1972	+	–	+Ø	...
Jugoslavia	0.01	++	+	++	++	++	++	(+) Hare
Turkey	0.59	+++	+	++	(+)	++	–	–

Zone III (Low Incidence, 0.6 – 3.0 cases/100,000 Pop. p.a.)

Great Britain	1.02	+ + +	+	–	–	–	–	–	Horse
Ireland	2.43	+	–	–	–	–	–	–	
France	0.95	+ + +	+ + Ø	+ + Ø	(+)	+ +	(+)	(–)	
USSR	2.40	+ + /	(+)	+ + Ø	+	+ +	+	+	Reindeer (*B. suis*)
									biotype 4
Hungary	1.11	+ +	– Ø	+ + Ø	+	–	+	:	
Albania	1.16	+ Ø	+ Ø	+ + Ø	(+)	+ +	+ + Ø	:	
Portugal	2.96	+ + +	+ +	: +	:	+ +	(+)	–	
Cyprus	0.60	–	–	+	–	+ +	–	–	

Zone IV (Moderate Incidence, 3.01 – 10.0 cases/100,000 Pop. p.a.)

Northern Ireland	5.13	(+)	–	–	–	–	–	
Scotland	6.00	+ + + +	–	–	–	+	–	
Italy	7.6	+ + +	+ +	+ +	+	+ +	+	

Zone V (High Incidence, above 10.0 cases/100,000 Pop. p.a.)

Spain	18.51	+ + + +	(+)	+ + +	+ + /	+ + +	+	Dog
Malta	15.66	+ + + + +	+ + + +	–	+ + + +	+	Horse
						+		
Greece	21.46	+ +	+ +	:	+ +	–	Horse
						+ +	+	Donkey
							+	Mule

3.1.2.3 Zone III: With Low Grade Brucellosis Frequency (0.6–3.0 Cases per 100,000 Inhabitants per Year). This zone includes countries as large as Great Britain, France, USSR, Hungary and Poland with more than 10 million inhabitants each.

Bovine Brucellosis in Zone III. These are countries with varying starting conditions as far as size of country, the number of inhabitants and the level of industrialization are concerned. In many cases intensive campaigns against bovine brucellosis were begun only a few years ago, and the organisation of the control programme varied greatly. For economic reasons some countries, like Great Britain, Northern Ireland and Greece – in contrast with the remaining northern and western European countries – tried at first to curtail the high rate of initial incidence by vaccinating calves with S 19 live vaccines. Only when investigations had shown conclusively that after years of vaccination a herd infection rate of below 10% and an individual infection rate of not more than 3% had been achieved, did the test and slaughter method find acceptance too in the last phase of elimination. Unfortunately this approach not only rather prolonged the overall duration of the operation but also gave rise to the necessity of distinguishing between samples affected by vaccination and those of genuine infection – which is not always easy for laboratory-technical reasons.

Countries which managed without the vaccination of calves tended to be in a position to announce brucellosis eradication earlier. Besides vaccinations, modern forms of animal husbandry (feed lots, pure milking herds), and the annual purchases of stock from a variety of herds have created fresh difficulties in the final elimination of bovine brucellosis in recent years, especially in Great Britain.[2]

Brucella melitensis of Sheep and Goats in Zone III. This appears, if at all, almost always among both these animals species at the same time and with similar force. Thus it still presents a low to medium grade problem for France, USSR, Albania, Portugal and Cyprus.

France and USSR are presently making great efforts to "control" brucellosis in sheep and goats by using Rev. 1 and H 38 live vaccine for lambs. Cyprus is on the way to becoming free from brucellosis in its flocks of sheep and goats and its cattle herds by applying the test and slaughter method (Polydorou 1979).

B. suis Brucellosis of Pigs in Zone III. In the endemic Zone III Great Britain, Ireland and Cyprus have so far been free from *B. suis* infections. Sporadic frequency of occurrence has been reported in France and Portugal, a low grade one from the USSR and Albania, and a still medium grade one from Hungary. All these countries apply the test and slaughter method.

Other Domestic and Wild Animals. Great Britain has reported cases of *B. abortus* in horses. Typical for brucella infections among domesticated and wild reindeer (caribou, *Rangifer tarandus, L.*) in the northern Siberian tundra is the appearance of its own biotype – *B. suis biotype 4* – which seems to be specific to this animal species. Man as a hunter and exploiter of the reindeer, and

---

2 According to a statement of the Minister of Agriculture, Mr. Peter Walker (The Times, 23rd of October 1981), Britain was declared free of brucellosis of cattle at 22nd of October 1981.

wolves as carnivores, had evidently been infected by the same *B. suis* biotype. Control measures which proceed similarly to those applied to cattle are very difficult to carry out under local conditions and the way of life of eskimos and reindeer, since one must accept an established natural focus among wild reindeer.

3.1.2.4 Zone IV: Medium Grade Frequency of Brucellosis Occurrence in Europe

Northern Europe. In two countries, Scotland and Northern Ireland, *B. abortus* brucellosis among cattle is the cause of a medium grade rate of incidence in man. Northern Ireland has, however, succeeded in reducing it to a merely sporadic occurrence. The rise in the case incidence rate may by attributed partly to improved diagnostic methods.

Southern Europe. Italy, like France, borders on the Mediterranean Sea. The large number of in part highly infected animal reservoirs make it impossible to achieve a rapid elimination of animal – and thus of human – brucellosis. With 7.6 cases per 100,000 inhabitants a year Italy heads the list in this endemic zone. Potential animal reservoirs in the north are mostly cattle (*Brucella abortus*), in the rest of the country, and especially in Sicily, sheep (*B. abortus, B. melitensis*), goats (*B. melitensis*) and pigs (*B. suis*), and all of the former suffer from a medium grade incidence of brucellosis infection. In Italy, cattle, sheep and goats are vaccinated against brucellosis (FAO 1974).

3.1.2.5 Zone V: High Grade Frequency of Incidence in Man

Southern Europe. Only three countries on the Mediterranean coasts appear in this category: Spain, Malta and Greece. In all of them *Brucella abortus* occurs in cattle and sheep, *B. melitensis* in sheep and goats. *B. ovis* has been reported in Spain, *B. suis* only in Spain and Greece. In Spain and Greece cattle, sheep and goats are vaccinated against brucellosis.

Other domesticated animals. In Spain dogs and horses, in Greece horses, donkeys and mules, were found to be infected with *Brucella abortus*. They are to be regarded as subsidiary hosts in the same biocoenosis, but can constitute a considerable health risk to man, especially where it is a matter of abscess forming infections among the equides.

3.2 Brucellosis Incidence in Africa

In screening the available literature brucellosis has been reported from

37/49   countries in man
41/49   countries in cattle with *B. abortus*
17/49   countries in sheep with *B. abortus*
28/49   countries in goats with *B. melitensis*
23/49   countries in sheep with *B. melitensis*
 9/49   countries in sheep with *B. ovis*
 8/49   countries in swine with *B. suis*
 5/49   countries in other domestic animals with unknown *B.* species
 6/49   countries in game animal species

1/49   countries reported brucellosis in man but not in animals

3/49   countries reported to be free of brucellosis at all, i.e. Mauritius, Madagascar and former Spanish Sahara

4/49   countries do either not report on brucellosis, i.e. Equat. Guinea, Benin,
and Cape Verde Islands, or only on brucellosis in man and goats but
not in cattle, i.e. Liberia.

Regarding the recognition of brucellosis by regular testing, already 25/49
(51.0%) of the African countries test regularly for bovine brucellosis, 7 (14.3%)
for ovine, 6 (12.2%) for caprine and 1 (2%) for equine brucellosis (i.e. in Chad)
(FAO 1974; answers to questionnaire).

About reporting on human brucellosis very little is known. Because of the
difficulty in the clinical diagnosis in animals, lack of facilities and setting of
other disease priorities brucellosis has been declared a scheduled disease in veterinary by-laws only in 25/49 (51.0%) African countries. 15/49 (30.6%) reported
brucellosis not to be a scheduled disease, for 9/49 (18.4%) countries no information was available.

Regular reporting as a scheduled disease of brucellosis on

b*	bo	bc	bs	boc	bocs	-brucellosis in
6	3	1	1	9	5	African countries

Legend: * b = bovine, o = ovine, c = caprine, s = swine

3.2.1 Bovine Brucellosis in Africa. Areas without any information on bovine
brucellosis have become scarce. A lot more investigations in the veterinary field
have filled the gap of information since 1959. With the exception of the two islands, Madagascar and Mauritius, which appear to be brucellosis-free, and the
countries Benin, Liberia, Equatorial Guinea, which did not report, there are 44
of 49 African countries with a greater or lesser degree of incidence of bovine
brucellosis. Summarizing the reports one can observe a high degree of incidence
in a ring of countries situated within the wet and dry savanna and tropical
rain forest zone around the Congo Forest area in West, Central and East Africa.
These countries in the savanna area also carry the main burden of cattle stock
in Africa.

This ring or "epicentre" of high brucellosis incidence is followed by another
ring of countries with a moderate or only low/sporadic incidence in the south,
west (except Mali) and north (except Morocco) of the continent.

Factors Influencing the Bovine Brucellosis Incidence

Climatic Factors. Thienpont et al. (1958) have shown that the local
microclimatic change caused by altitude may play a role in the degree of
incidence in bovine brucellosis. Working in Rwanda, East Africa, they found a
prevalence rate of between 7.8−19.8% at an altitude of 1500−1700 meters
above sea level where the climate is warm and humid; but the prevalence rate
dropped on the same mountain within herds of about the same size to less than
2% at an altitude of 1900 meters where the climate is humid and cold.

Herd-Size and Management. Hoffmann and El Sawah (1969) in Tanzania proved the old epizootological rule of "small herd-low incidence, large herd-high incidence of brucellosis" (Table 6).

But our own investigations in Uganda (Thimm and Wundt 1976) have shown that this rule can only be applied when comparing herds of the same breed within the same area and under the same climatic and management conditions.

Thus one can expect that with the introduction of modern cattle husbandry and ranching methods, mainly with the buying in of cattle of unknown origin, brucellosis will become a major disease problem in developing countries.

Table 6. Herd-size, management and infection rate

Herd-size	Management	Ownership	Infection rate
20 h/c	sedative extensive individual grazing	private	3.8%
20 – 200 h/c	sedative extensive communal grazing	private	12.2%
200 h/c	sedative semi-intensive	Government	29.7%

3.2.2 Brucellosis Incidence in Sheep and Goats. The Map of Brucellosis in Africa gives information on the occurrence and incidence of brucellosis in sheep in 19 countries and in goats in 25 countries.

Comparing the prevalence rates reported with that of bovine brucellosis it is very interesting that the group of small ruminants first domesticated by man, the sheep and the goat, show very uniformly a low/sporadic degree of incidence throughout the continent, although with a few exceptions. In Niger and Upper Volta, Gidel et al. (1972) using the Milk Ring Test in addition to the Serum Agglutination Test (SAT) received much higher prevalence rates than with the individual SAT alone. If taking the herd as the epizootiological parameter of prime importance one could calculate a 5–10 times higher incidence rate than hitherto known for the national goat and sheep herds.

B. ovis in Sheep in Africa. B. ovis isolations have been reported from sheep in:
Egypt, Tunisia and Mauretania in the North,
Mali, Niger and Nigeria in the West,
Kenya and Rhodesia in the East and Mozambique and the South African Republic in the south of Africa (see Table 7).

3.2.3 B. suis in Swine in Africa. Available figures about *B. suis* in swine greatly depend on 2 factors:
a) the economic interest in pig breeding and pig diseases
b) the scientific interest in pig diseases and the reporting of brucellosis in swine.

As Arab countries on the African continent do not lay emphasis on pig breeding for religious reasons, one should expect reports mainly from south of the Sahara. Indeed, 8 countries, situated in the West (Mali, Senegal, Sierra Leone and Nigeria), Central (Congo Rep., Zaire) and South-East Africa (Zimbabwe, Mozambique) appear to have a problem with brucellosis in swine. This does

Table 7. Incidence of human brucellosis in Africa (reported cases per 100,000 P.p.a.) in comparison with animal brucellosis in the reported countries (Period 1968–1975)

Inc.: free	sporadic, 0 – 0.59					low, 0.6 – 3.0					moderate, 3.01 – 10.0				high, above 10.0				
Reported animal brucellosis in	Country	b.	o.	c.	s.[1]	Country	b.	o.	c.	s.	Country	b.	o. c. s.		Country	b.	o.	c.	s.
North Africa																			
Span. Sahara	Egypt	++	+	+	?	Ethiopia	++	+	+	?	–				–				
	Algeria	+++	++	+	?	Libya	+	?	?	–	–				–				
	Morocco	++++	+	+	–	Mauretania	++	+	+	?	–				–				
	Tunesia	+++	++	+++	?	Sudan	++++	+	+	–	–				–				
East Africa																			
	Zambia	++	+	?	?	Kenya	++	+	+	–	Tanzania	++	+ + ?		Terr. Affars	?	?	?	
	Somalia	++	+	+	–	Uganda	+++	+	+	?	–				–				
						Rwanda	++++	++	+	–	–				–				
						Burundi	++++	++	–	–	–				–				
						Malawi	+++	–	–	–	–				–				
South Africa																			
Madagaskar[2]	Lesotho	+	?	–	?	Angola	++	–	–	–	–				–				
Mauritius	Mozambique	+++	+	+	+	Botswana	+++	++	++	?	–				–				
	S. Africa	+++	+	+++	–	–					–				–				
West Africa																			
	Liberia	?	+	?	?	Gambia	++	+	?	?	Zaire	++++	+ + +		Nigeria	+++	++	++	+
	Mali	++++	++	?	+	Congo	++	+	–	+	–				–				
	Chad	++++	++	+	?	Ghana	+++	–	–	?	–				–				
						Niger	+++	++++	+++	?	–				–				
						Up. Volta	+++	+++	++	+	–				–				
						Senegal	++	++	++	+	–				–				
						Swaziland	+++	–	?	?	–				–				

1 b: bovine; o: ovine; c: caprine; s: swine brucellosis
2 Dog serologically positive

not exclude that swine brucellosis does not occur in the other African countries not reporting unless it has been proven by careful survey testing.

3.2.4 Brucellosis in the African Wild Fauna.

6 African countries reported so far on the serological and/or bacteriological proof of brucellosis in the wild fauna, i.e. Zimbabwe, the South African Republic, Zambia, Tanzania, Uganda and the Chad. From the hundreds of wild animals screened the following prevalence rates were received (in ascending order): 3.2% in the Chad, 8.3% in the R.S.A., 10.5% in Rhodesia, 11.1% in Tanzania, 23.1% in Uganda. Proof of brucellosis was also obtained in 2 eland antelopes grazing with a herd of aborting goats in Zambia.

The following herbivorous game species appear frequently on the list of positive animal species:

The eland (*Taurotragus oryx, L*), African buffalo (*Syncerus caffer, L*), hippopotamus (*Hippopotamus amphibius, L*), zebra (*Equus burchelli, L*), wildbeest (*Connochaetes taurinus, L*), impala (*Aepyceros melampus, L*), waterbuck (*Kobus defassa, L*), and bushbuck (*Tragelaphus scriptus, L*).

To these herbivorous game species comes the group of wild carnivores and scavengers living on the game, like spotted hyena (*Crocuta crocuta, L*), wild dogs (*Lycaon pictus, L*), black-backed jackal (*Canis mesomelas, L*) and the lion (*Panthera leo, L*). With the exception of the eland, waterbuck and bushbuck, all the other herbivorous species appear often in great numbers at a time, thus facilitating the spread of *brucella* via aborted foetuses, foetal membranes and vaginal discharges to the pasture and other susceptible animals.

With 81% (21/26) of the herbivorous and 42% (5/12) of the carnivorous species of wild animals screened carrying antibodies to *brucella* antigen one can expect that closed natural infection cycles must exist without further contact with domestic animals. But this needs further evidence (Thimm and Wundt 1976).

It is interesting to note the high prevalence of *brucella* antibodies in water fowls like ducks and geese found in the Chad. This points to the importance which surface water has within the natural infection cycle of game and domestic animals.

Cross-infections between game and domestic animals can be accepted in the pandemic East African countries. *B. melitensis biotype 1* has been isolated from an impala in Tanzania (Schiemann and Staak 1971) and from sheep and goats in Kenya (Philpott 1970). *B. abortus biotype 3*, the main *B. abortus* biotype found in the indigenous cattle in East Africa (Rollinson 1962; Hummel and Staak 1974) was also found in the East African buffalo (Schiemann and Staak 1971) and *B. abortus biotype 1*, usually found in the exotic cattle herds in East and South Africa (Thimm 1967; Mansvelt 1975), was also isolated from a waterbuck in Zimbabwe (Condy and Vickers 1972) and from the African buffalo in the Kruger National Park in the South African Republic (OIE, 1969).

The potential and direct danger of game animal brucellosis for man in Africa was proven in 1971 by the close cooperation between a medical and two veterinary doctors in Tanzania. After Young had isolated *B. melitensis biotype 1* from an infected game guard who had contracted brucellosis during a large anti-tsetse-game cropping scheme in northern Tanzania, Schiemann and Staak (1971) succeeded in isolating the same strain from an impala of the same area.

Thus, although modern animal husbandry methods with fencing has been introduced to a marginal extent *in African countries close contacts between domestic and game animals and man are likely to remain and to maintain the brucellosis infection cycles also in future.*

3.2.5 Human Brucellosis in Africa. Human brucellosis, as the geomedical survey has shown, is known to exist in 37 of the 49 (75.5%) African countries. The incidence is low/sporadic on the major part of the continent, especially in the low-rainfall-zones in the north, east and south, areas which are mainly utilized for goat and sheep keeping (see Table 7).

Keeping in mind the large number of animal foci present in Africa one should expect most of its countries to be ridden with brucellosis. The more one is surprised about the reported low/sporadic incidence almost throughout the continent. As an exception Tanzania and Zaire report a moderate, Nigeria and the Territory of Affars and Issars a high incidence. Moreover tests to pin-point the major animal group acting as disease reservoir for brucellosis have pointed to the small ruminant group of sheep and goats.

Thus Collard (1962) has tested 3,232 human sera in Nigeria with two different antigens. 26.4% reacted more to the *B. abortus,* 31.4% to the *melitensis* antigen. But as the antigen relationship between *B. abortus* and *B. melitensis* antigen is very close one should regard these results with caution. Cox (1966) tried to clarify the epidemiological situation in the traditional nomadic tribes in Karamoja, north-east Uganda. He reported that 72.5% of the clinically positive brucellosis cases gave higher serotiters with *B. melitensis* and only 11% with *B. abortus* antigen, 16.5% had equally high titres. These herdsmen live largely on cattle milk and blood, their huge herds consist mainly of cattle with a few sheep, goats and donkeys. *Brucella* strain isolations, the only acceptable epidemiological method for comparative bacteriological studies, were performed by Wright (1953) in Kenya, who revealed that *brucella* infections in Africans were predominantly caused by *B. melitensis* but in Europeans almost exclusively by *B. abortus.* Oomen (1976) retesting this arrived at the same results regarding African brucella carriers.

It appears from these results that even for the nomadic herdsmen with the large cattle and small sheep and goat herds moving away in the transhumance from the daily grazing grounds the small ruminants present the main risk to health. For it is not so much the number of animals of a certain species but the human habits and customs of keeping sheep and goats within the compound and even within the same house of his family, as well as the drinking of raw goats' milk and eating mainly goat and sheep meat and milkproducts, that present a larger risk of infection to the human population in African countries than the often large cattle herds which are kept away from the house. Yet the whole spectrum of the human-animal-disease relationship is so big that one cannot generalize.

3.3 Brucellosis in the Americas

North America has almost reached the aim of freedom from brucellosis, whereas Latin America is still in the midst of a strong animal brucellosis control and eradication programme in order to reduce the largely sporadic occurrence of human brucellosis (0.0–0.59 cases per 100,000 inhabitants per year) still further. A low-grade incidence (0.6–3.0 cases per 100,000 inhabitants per year) was still found in Mexico, and a medium-grade one (3.01–10.0 cases per 100,000 inhabitants per year) in Peru and Argentina. A summary of the reported cases of brucellosis per year is given in Table 9 and Fig. 2 (see special

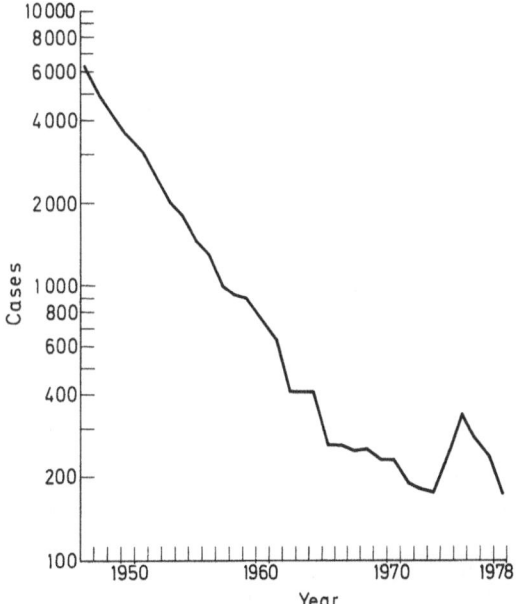

Fig. 2. Human brucellosis, United States of America, Period 1947–1978

map 1 at the back of plate 3). One should remember at this point that we are mapping only reported cases. According to this, the U.S.A., after 15 years of intensive measures against brucellosis, dealing with an annual average of 223 cases, which results in a case rate of 0.10 per 100,000 inhabitants, are statistically now well placed. Nothing can be said about the quality of the reporting discipline and the individual reports. In many countries neither the actual infection rate nor the "grey" figure are known.

The overall review of case reports shows, however, that in the selected period 1970–77, nine out of twenty one countries did already provide an annual report, and 19 out of 21 did so at least every second year. Four countries stood out especially, thanks to their high incidence rates, which amounted to more than 100 per annum; these were Argentina, U.S.A., Mexico and Peru. But, if the assumption is correct, one should regard this high incidence rate more as an indication of a high reporting discipline than of a true difference in the brucellosis problem within the American countries. Therefore one cannot realistically com-

Table 8. Brucellosis in the Americas in man and animals. (Period 1970–1977)

Country	Human cases per 100,000 Pop. p.a.	Cattle		Sheep		Goat	Swine	Other dom. animals	Wild animals
		B. ab.	*B. mel.*	*B. mel.*	*B. ovis*	*B. mel.*	*B. suis*		
North America and Mexico									
Canada	0.11+	(+)	—	(—)	—	—	+	Horse, Dog+	Reindeer
U.S.A.	0.10	+/	(+)	+	+	(+)	+		Elk
Mexico	1.16++	++++	?	+	?	+++	+		Moose, Horse+ Bison, Dog+
Central America and the Caribic									
Belize (Brit. Hond.)	...?	++	(—)	(—)	(—)	(—)	(—)	:	:
Guatemala	...?	+++	(+)	(—)	(—)	:	:	:	:
El Salvador	0.05 +	+	—	?	(—)	?	?	:	—
Honduras	0.10	++	(—)	—	—	—	?	:	—
Nicaragua	...?	+++	(—)	—	—	:	—	:	:
Costa Rica	0.30	+++	:	:	:	:	:	:	:
Panama	0.25	++	:	:	:	:	?	:	:
Bermudas	...?	+/	:	(—)	(—)	—	:	:	:
Bahamas	...?	+ + +	(—)	(—)	(—)	(—)	(—)	:	(—)
Cuba	0.19	+ +	(+)	(+)	(—)	(—)	—	:	:
Jamaica	...+	(+)	(—)	(—)	(—)	—	—	:	:
Haiti	...?	++	—	: +	:	—	—	:	—
Dom. Rep.	0.02	++	—	+	—	—	?	:	:
Barbados	0.25+	—	—	—	—	—	—	:	—
Trinidad a. Tob.	...		—	—	—	—	—	:	
Am. Virg. Islands	...	—	—	—	—	—	—	:	:
South America									
Argentina	5.0+++	+++Ø	?	—	++++Ø	++++Ø	+++Ø	Dog+Horse+	Buffalo+
Brazil	...?	++	:	(—)	+++Ø	mel—ab+suis+	++	Horse+Dog+	:
Chile	0.09+	+++/	?	(—)	(+)	+Ø/	++	Dog+	:
Paraguay	0.19+	+	:	:	:	—	:	:	—
Uruguay	0.03+	++	:	:	:	—	:	Horse+	:
Peru	5.36+++	+	(—)+	++	++	+ +	(—)	Alpaca+	(—)
Ecuador	...+	+++	+	—	?	++	+++	:	:
Columbia	0.18+	+++	—	?	—	—	(+)+	:	—
Venezuela	0.04	++.	:	?	(—).	?	++.	:	:
Guyana	?								

pare the reported case figures between the countries. A synoptic presentation shows which animal reservoirs are responsible for these high annual numbers of cases (see Table 8).

3.3.1 Brucellosis in North America. With an annual incidence rate of 0.11 or 0.10 per 100,000 inhabitants respectively, *Canada* and the *U.S.A.* are now very close to the aim of being free from brucellosis (0.01 cases per 100,000 inhabitants per year). The chief animal reservoirs are cattle and pigs. By virtue of their jobs workers in slaughterhouses, veterinarians and farmers are especially at risk.

In *Canada* further animal reservoirs were observed in horses and dogs (*B. abortus* and *B. suis*), in the U.S.A. in dogs (*B. canis*), sheep (*B. ovis* and *B. abortus*), and occasionally in goats (*B. melitensis*).

Wild animals, such as the bison (*Bison bison, L*) and the wapiti stag (*Cervus canadensis, L*) may be independent primary as well as cattle-dependent secondary natural reservoirs of brucellosis (Choquette et al. 1978, Corner and Connell, 1958). The moose (*Alces alces, L*) does not, however, appear to be a natural carrier of brucellosis (Hudson, 1980). *B. suis biotype 1* frequently occurs in wild boars in Florida (53 per cent sero-positive reactions by 95 trapped animals, 9/9 bacteriologically positive; Becker et al. 1978). The American desert wood rat (*Neotoma lepida, Thomas*) was found to have its own brucellosis species (*B. neotomae*).

Both these countries − Canada as well as the U.S.A. − are free from melitensis brucellosis in man. However, there is occasionally evidence of melitensis brucellosis in herds of goats. The reason for this is unknown. The elimination of the disease is achieved by slaughter of the complete herd.

In *Alaska, northern Canada* and *Siberia,* wild and domesticated reindeer (*Rangifer tarandus granti* and *R. tarandi groenlandicus, L*), together with eskimos and predators (wolf, bear, fox) that feed on them, were found to have their own *B. suis* biotype 4. Transmission to man probably takes place by direct contact, as with cattle, or orally through the consumption of raw or undercooked meat (see Special Maps 3 and 4 on the back of Map 3).

Mexico. With 1.16 cases of infection per 100,000 inhabitants per annum, the rate of incidence is about ten times as high as in the U.S.A. and Canada. Cattte (*B. abortus* ++++) and goats (*B. melitensis* +++) are regarded as the main animal reservoir. There are also some sporadic incidences of melitensis brucellosis among sheep, and of *B. suis* among pigs. In Mexico brucellosis constitutes a health problem of medium dimension, which in turn assumes the role of a major economic problem. Besides reports of infections the control measures include the test-and-slaughter method among cattle and the vaccination of calves and lambs.

3.3.2 Brucellosis in Central America and the Caribbean Islands. The three island states of Bermuda, the Bahamas and Trinadad and Tobago are reportedly free from brucellosis in man. Occasional cases of bovine brucellosis are said to occur in the Bahamas and Bermuda.

Table 9. Human brucellosis – reported cases in Latin America 1970–1977

Country	1970	1971	1972	1973	1974	1975	1976	1977	Total	Av. cases/year rep.	Population i. 1,000	Brucellosis rate/100,000 Inh.
Argentina	1,071	1,119	1,114	986	1,123	1,293	1,569	1,727	10,002	1,250	25,000	5.0
Bolivia	...	...	1	3	1	2	...	...	7	1	5,000	0.02
Brazil	...	...	...	...	...	...	...	...				
Canada	31	8	17	8	27	27	38	39	195	24	22,000	0.11
Chile	1	4	4	...	...	51	...	...	60	15	10,000	0.15
Colombia	35	42	31	25	69	...	...	...	202	40	23,000	0.17
Costa Rica	11	1	...	6	5	7	6	...	36	6	2,000	0.30
Cuba	11	21	9	18	10	34	14	...	117	17	9,000	0.19
El Salvador	...	6	—	—	1	...	...	...	7	4	3,000	0.13
Honduras	5	2	1	3	4	4	—	1	20	3	3,000	0,10
Mexico	612	777	761	735	477	550	469	...	4,381	626	54,000	1,16
Panama	3	—	—	1	4	...	5	7	20	4	1,000	0.40
Paraguay	1	15	—	3	—	...	...	...	19	6	2,000	0.30
Peru	1,118	1,284	822	607	501	424	546	610	5,912	739	14,000	5.28
Uruguay	—	3	1	—	...	1	...	—	5	2	3,000	0.07
U.S.A.	213	171	196	202	197	310	282	216	1,787	223	216,332	0.10
Venezuela	7	4	11	...	...	2	—	...	28	6	11,000	0.05

— no cases reported
.... no data

Lit.: 1. Boletin Informativo 1978, Centro Panamericano de Zoonoses WHO Buenos Aires, Argentina
2. WHO-Center, Geneva
3. FAO/WHO Animal Health Year Book, 1974

The states of Belize, Guatemala, Nicaragua, Haiti and the American Virgin Islands did not issue any reports on human brucellosis. Those concerning infections in animal herds were of a very fragmentary nature.

In Central America and in the Caribbean Islands cattle appear to constitute the only animal reservoir. This permits the conclusion to be drawn that cattle-buying has been responsible for the introduction and distribution of brucellosis in historic times. However, more detailed investigations might well result − even here − in some adjustments to this picture. There have been reports on the sporadic occurrence of melitensis brucellosis among sheep from Barbados, of *B. abortus* brucellosis among sheep in El Salvador and Cuba, and of *B. suis* brucellosis from Panama and Cuba. The latter is always eliminated by the test-and-slaughter method. Considering the initial situation, Cuba has achieved good results throughout its campaign against brucellosis.

3.3.3 Brucellosis in South America. The situation of brucellosis in South America presents a much more strongly marked picture. From the point of view of public health and the economy it is still *the* most important zoonosis in South America (Szyfres, 1973). The economic losses for Brazil and Argentina in 1972 alone were calculated to amount to US $ 400 and 108 million respectively. These are countries which are just beginning to take measures against brucellosis. In the U.S.A. where losses of US $ 100 million were still registered as recently as 1947, it was reckoned in 1972 − that is 15 years after the start of a co-ordinated and strong anti-brucellosis campaign − that losses were below US $ 10 million. The difference must be regarded as an annual contribution to the national income. In 1965, as a result of human brucellosis, Argentina's 25 million inhabitants had, moreover, to sustain losses calculated at 595 million US dollars per 1000 patients. In this figure the considerable losses resulting from lost working hours and production, as well as the costs of treatment and rehabilitation, were summed up. The number of brucellosis cases registered in Argentina rose from 1114 in 1972 to 1727 in 1977 (Table 9).

So too, in South America the epidemiological spectrum ranges from "free" (Surinam, French Guiana) to high-grade incidence of brucellosis (Argentina, Peru). In the cases of Brazil and Ecuador no annual incidence rates have been published. Considering, however, that the initial epizootiological situation is very similar to that of Argentina, a similar incidence rate must also be assumed there.

Not only does the economic state of development vary among the individual countries of South America, but so also does the distribution of individual brucella species; indeed, even the individual brucella biotypes (as the results of strain typification will confirm) (Tables 10 and 11).

Brucellosis Control Measures. According to the magnitude of the infection rate among the herds and single animals (cattle, sheep, goats, pigs and alpacas) different control methods are applied. Apart from Guyana, all these countries have begun their campaigns by vaccinating calves with S 19 live vaccine for periods of several years with the aim of building up a high degree of immunity protection against re-infection; but Brazil, Peru, Venezuela and Colombia have already gone further and introduced the test-and-slaughter method among

Table 10. Pattern of distribution of Brucella species

Brucella species:	B. abortus B. melitensis B. suis	B. abortus B. melitensis	B. abortus B. suis	B. abortus
Country:	Argentina Brasil Chile Ecuador Guiana	Peru	Colombia Venezuela	Paraguay Uruguay

cattle. Because of the high initial level of infection in Ecuador and Peru, *B. melitensis* brucellosis is first tackled by vaccinating lambs and kids with Rev. 1 live vaccine. Additional test-and-slaughter programmes for sheep are carried out in Peru, as for goats in Chile, and against *B. suis* brucellosis in swine in Brazil and Venezuela.

Regulations in respect of quarantine for imported – or, as the case may be, for brucella-positive-cattle, sheep, goats and pigs are only in force in Venezuela, and for cattle, sheep and pigs in Colombia too.

Distribution Pattern of Brucella Species and Biotypes in the Countries of South America and the Caribbean Islands. The best epidemiological evidence for a certain distribution pattern of brucella species is their typification and classification according to criteria of bacteriology, geography and animal species. Since 1971 th s has been made possible by the regular publications from C. Carcia Carillo et al. (1971) of the Panamerican Centre for Zoonosis of the WHO, Ramos Mejia, Argentina (Table 11).

Particularities of Distribution in the Host. Table 11 only lists the typifiable strains of *brucella*, arranged according to host and country of isolation.

The 794 brucella strains which were collected and evaluated over the period 1965–77 at the WHO centre at Ramos Mejia belong to the following species:

Br. species	Strains typed		Isolated from man	
	N	%	N	%
B. abortus	324	40.8	27	8.3
B. melitensis	298	37.5	252	84.6
B. suis	101	12.7	48	47.5
B. ovis	68	8.6	–	–
B. canis	3	0.4	–	–
Total	794	100.0	327	100.0

B. abortus. This species has so far been isolated in man (27 strains), in cattle (279 strains), in sheep (1 strain) and in pigs (1 strain), but *not* in goats. Biotype 1 dominated (with 34%) and was followed by biotype 4 (4.6%), biotype 2 (1.5%) and biotype 3 (0.8%).

Table 11. Brucella species and biotypes isolated in the Americas and Caribbean (Panamerican Zoonoses Center, WHO, Informativo Bulletin, 1965–1977)

	Strains typed	B. abortus				B. melitensis			B. suis	B. ovis	B. canis
		Bio 1	Bio 2	Bio 3	Bio 4	Bio 1	Bio 2	Bio 3	Bio 1		
Host species											
Man	327	26	1			245	5	2	48		
Cattle	282	226	11	6	36				3		
Sheep	75	1				3			3	68	
Goats	49					40			9		
Swine	37	1							36		
Other domestic and wild animals	24	16				3			2		3
Countries											
Argentina	220	82	1		9	29			51	45	2
Brazil	57	23	9	6					19	12	
Chile	95	47			11	14	5		6		
Colombia	81	69	1		1				10		
Cuba	31	26			3				2		
Ecuador	8	1			6				1		
Honduras	1								1		
Mexico	160	3				148		2	7		
Peru	114	9				100				4	1
Uruguay	10	4	1							7	
Venezuela	9	4							4		
Nicaragua	8	2			6						
Total	794	270	12	6	36	291	5	2	101	68	3
%	100.0	34.0	1.5	0.8	4.6	37.0	0.6	0.3	12.7	8.7	0.4

Isolation from other animal species: fox (10 strains), ferret (1 strain) and horse (5 strains).

B. melitensis. In South America and the Caribbean Islands *B. melitensis* is the main agent for brucellosis in man. Biotype 1 (74.9%) dominates and is followed by biotype 2 (1.5%) and biotype 3 (0.6%). *Goats were the main reservoir hosts.* Sheep (3 strains in Argentina) and alpacas (3 strains in Peru) functioned only as subsidiary hosts. Strangely enough, the biotypes 2 (in Chile with 5 strains) and 3 (in Mexico, with 2 strains) isolated in man have so far not recurred in any host animal in the countries of the Americas. Tourism or the importation of infected milk products may have played a role here.

B. suis. Accounting for only 12.7% of the total isolations, *B. suis* strains are relatively rare in the overall collective. Nevertheless, strains isolated from man and totalling 48/101 contributed the largest share of a single host in it. This is certainly a question of search for and preselection of cases according to clinical and professional viewpoints. Besides pigs (with 36 strains), the only other surprising frequency occurred among goats (9 strains), whereas incidence among cattle (3 strains), sheep (3 strains), hares (1 strain) and dogs (1 strain) was rare.

Particularities in Geographical Distribution

B. abortus.
Biotype 1. evidence in 11 out of 12 countries under investigation.
Biotype 2. large numbers in Brazil, fewer in Argentina, Colombia and Venezuela.
Biotype 3. only in Brazil.
Biotype 4. large numbers in Chile, Argentina and Ecuador, but rarely isolated in Colombia and Cuba.

B. melitensis.
Biotype 1. evidence in 4 out of 12 countries under investigation, such as Argentina and Chile, and in great numbers in Mexico and Peru.
Biotype 2. found only in Chile.
Biotype 3. found only in Mexico

B. suis. Biotype 1. evidence in 9 out of 12 countries under investigation. Very frequent in Argentina, Brazil and Colombia, but less so in Chile and Mexico and sporadic in Cuba, Ecuador and Honduras.

B. ovis: To date isolated only in 4 out of 12 countries under investigation; frequently in Argentina and Chile, less frequently in Uruguay and Peru.

B. canis: Following its original isolation in the U.S.A., this new brucella species has meanwhile been confirmed in dogs in Argentina and Peru.

4 The Incidence of Brucellosis in Asia, Australia and Oceania

It was not possible to compile a picture of the distribution of brucellosis and the Brucella species for the remaining countries of the Asian and Australian continents and Oceania which was even approximately complete. The statements on occurrence among domestic animals vary greatly – evidently in accordance with their varying economic significance. For this reason an exact account of the distribution must await further investigations.

4.1 Asia

A summary of the results up to now are given in Table 12. Only 9 out of 38 countries have so far supplied exact data on cases in man during the period 1968–74 (Lebanon, Israel, Iraq, Iran, Kuwait, Sri Lanka, the Khmer Republic, Laos and Indonesia). External influences, too, make themselves felt in the reporting system of the health services. For the Khmer Republic at least a considerable "grey" figure is to be assumed. Out of 38 countries

17 reported the occurrence of *B. abortus* in man
11 reported the occurrence of *B. melitensis* in man
30 reported the occurrence of *B. abortus* in cattle
 8 reported the occurrence of *B. abortus* in sheep
15 reported the occurrence of *B. melitensis* in sheep
 4 reported the occurrence of *B. ovis* in sheep
15 reported the occurrence of *B. melitensis* in goats
11 reported the occurrence of brucellosis in other domestic and wild animals

Other animal species		*Brucella* species	*Brucella* incidence
Iran	dog	*B. melitensis*	+
	buffalo	*B. abortus*	+
Pakistan	buffalo	*B. abortus*	+
India	dog	*B. melitensis*	+
	buffalo	*B. melitensis, B. abortus*	++
Bangladesh	buffalo	*B. abortus*	++
Thailand	buffalo	*B. abortus*	++
Vietnam	horse	*B. abortus*	+
Mongolia	camel	*B. melitensis*	++
Japan	dog	*B. canis*	+
Philippines	horse	*B. abortus*	++++
Indonesia	buffalo	*B. abortus*	++++

Table 12. Brucellosis incidence in Asia (period 1968–74)

Country	Reported hum. cases per 100,000 Pop. p.a.	Man B. ab.	Man B. mel.	Cattle B. ab.	Sheep B. ab.	Sheep B. mel.	Sheep B. ov.	Goat B. mel.	Swine B. suis	Game and other dom. animals
Syrian A.R.	..	+	+	+	+	+	+	+	..	..
Lebanon	0.08	+	+	++	?	+	?	++	..	..
Israel	0.63	++	++	++	–	+	–	++	–	–
Jordan	..	?	?	–	–	+	–	+	–	–
Iraq	0.03	+	..	+	–	–	–	?	–	–
Iran	11.9	+++	+++	+++	?	?	..	+++	+++	Horse + Buffalo +
Afghanistan		+++	++	++	?	+++	+	+++	–	–
Pakistan		?	+	++	?	?	–	++	–	Buffalo +
Saudi Arab.		?	..	+	+	+	..	+	–	..
Yemen Ar. Rep.		?	..	+	–	..	..	..	..	..
Yemen P. Rep.		?	..	+	..	..	..	–	–	–
Unt. Ar. Emir.			..	+	?	?	?	?	–	–
Qatar		..	..	?	?	?	?	–	–	..
Bahrain		..	..	+	+	–	(–)	..	..	..
Kuwait	1.86	++	++	+++	?	(–)	?	(?)	(–)	–
Sri Lanka	0.16	+	..	+++	..	+	(–)	+	+	Dog + Buffalo + B. mel.
India		+	..	+++	++	+	+	–	+	–
Nepal		?	+	++	+	?	(+)	+	..	Buffalo + B. mel.
Bangladesh		?	?	++	..	+	?	+	..	..
Burma		?	?	+	–	+	–	+	+	Buffalo + B. ab.
Thailand		..	++	+	–	+	..	+	++++	..
Khmer Rep.	0.52	++	++	+	–	+	..	+	+	..
Laos P. Rep.	10.16	+++	++	++	?	+	..	..	+	..

Viet Nam	+	?	+	+	+	:	:	+	Horse + B. suis
China P. Rep.	:	++++	:+	:	:	:	:+	:	Camel + B. suis
Mongolia P. Rep.	:	?	++	++	:	++	?	:	
Macao	+	:	+++	:	:	:	-	:	
Hong Kong	+	:	+++	:	:	++	:	:	
Taiwan	-	-	+(+)	:	:	:	:(-)	:	
Korea	:	+	+	:	:	-	:(-)	:	Dog + B. canis
Japan	+	:	++	-	-	-	-	:	Horse +++
Philippines	?	:	++++	-	-	+	-	:	Buffalo +++
Indonesia	:	:	-	-	-	-	-	-	-
Port. Timor	?	:	-	?	-	-	-	-	-
Singapore	+	?	+	:	:	++++	:	+	
Malaysia (Sarawak)	?	:	-	:	:	+	:	:	
Malaysia (Sabah)	:	?	-	:	:	-	:	:	
Brunei	?	?	+	:	:	+	:	-	
Malaysia (Western)									

A particularly serious brucellosis problem is reported from the *Iran* (Sab-baghian and Nadim 1974). The provinces of Azerbaijan, Khorasan, Mazande-ran and Baluchistan are particularly affected. The *epicentre* is maintained by a large number of infected domestic host animals, such as cattle, buffaloes, sheep, pigs, dogs and horses, with man being most frequently infected by *B. melitensis.* In spite of years of efforts to control brucellosis, including reporting, tests, slaughtering and vaccination (calves with S. 19 and lambs with Rev. 1 live vac-cines) these activities have not succeeded in essentially reducing the number of infections in man. In the period from 1967 to 1971 an average of 3,350 cases have been reported each year.

A *second epicentre* is situated in the *India-Pakistan-Bangladesh-Sri Lanka re-gion.* Not only are cattle, sheep and goats – together with pigs and dogs in India – affected there, but a considerable number of large herds of water buffalo suf-fer from brucellosis as well.

A plethora of individual data makes it possible to present an overall picture of the distribution of brucellosis in India (Table 13).

A *third epicentre* appears to be situated in *Laos.* In 1964 and again in 1965 more than 300 cases were reported to the WHO from there. Unfortunately fur-ther reports have not been forthcoming. No information is available in the case of the *Peoples' Republic of China.* The adjacent states of Mongolia and Hong Kong, however, have a considerable brucellosis problem. It ought therefore to be assumed that China, too, is not free from brucellosis.

Investigations by Jezek et al. (1974) showed another *epicentre* of *B. meliten-sis* in the *Mongolian Peoples' Republic.* Here the infected and rather weak lambs, born in the wintry conditions of spring and taken to the shelter of tents by the nomads, are the main source of brucellosis infection, especially among children. Besides the cattle, sheep and goats as well as camels are regarded as animal reservoirs.

Table 13. Brucellosis incidence in India

	Man	Cattle	Buffalo	Goat	Sheep	Pig	Other
Kashmir Valley	+++	. . .	. . .	. . .	. . .	. . .	. . .
Punjab	+++	+[1]	+	+++*	+++*	+	dog
Delhi	+++	+++[2]	. . .	. . .	. . .	+	. . .
Ut. Pradesh	++	–	. . .	+	+	+	. . .
Bihar	+	+++	. . .	+	+	+	. . .
West Bengal	++	++++	+++	+	+	+	. . .
Assam	+	++	+	+	+	. . .	. . .
M. Pradesh	+	++	+	+	+	. . .	. . .
Orissa	+	+++	+	++	+	. . .	poultry
A. Pradesh	+	+++	+	+	+	. . .	. . .
Tamil N, Ma	+	+	+	+	+	. . .	. . .
Mysore	+	++++	+	+	+	. . .	. . .
Maharashtra	+	+++	++	+	+	++	. . .
Gujarat	+	++	+	+	+	. . .	. . .

1 Native cattle, privately owned
2 Cattle on Govt. farms
* Goats and sheep in Haryana (Punjab) infected with *B. mel.* and *B. abortus*

Indonesia is a state made up of 10,000 islands, but brucellosis occurrence is reported only in the larger ones.

Northern Sumatra	Buffalo	++++	man + *B. abortus?*
Java	Buffalo	+++	man + *B. abortus?*
Eastern Java		++++	
Western Irian	Buffalo	+++	man + *B. abortus?*
Jakarta	Pigs	+	man + *B. abortus, B. suis*

There is no *melitensis* brucellosis reported.

The same applies to the *Philippines.*

They report a low-grade occurrence of *B. abortus* brucellosis among cattle in the provinces of Butungus, Lunno, Masbate, Pangasinan and Cebu, with only sporadic incidence in the rest of the country, although there is a high-grade occurrence among horses; infection among pigs is sporadic, the agent being *B. suis.* Man is said to be only sporadically affected.

Returns from *Malaysia* (Sarawak) and *Thailand* showed a high rate of infection among pigs with *B. suis.*

The exceptions in the disease's general picture are *Korea* and *Japan.* Years of persistent control programmes, including the obligatory reporting of cases, as well as the test-and-slaughter method, have enabled both of them to eliminate brucellosis among domestic animals, and thus indirectly in man. Korea now reports only the odd case among cattle, and in Japan even these occur only among imported cattle undergoing quarantine.

After the discovery of the first cases of *B. canis* in dogs in Japan, however, the same was detected in man, which had been brought about − as in the U.S.A. − through close contact with dogs or as laboratory infections. However, they are rarities.

4.2 The Incidence of Brucellosis in Australia and Oceania (Table 14)

Reports from the fifth continent and the oceanian islands are favourable in respect of brucellosis distribution among man. Apart from one questionable occurrence of *Brucella melitensis* among goats in New Caledonia the entire Australia/Oceania region appears to be free from *B. melitensis* brucellosis. However, Australia and New Zealand still have a low-grade problem of cases of *B. abortus* in man, and French Polynesia even has a high-grade one; these are closely linked with assistance to infected cattle. A sporadic occurrence of swine brucellosis is reported in Australia, New Zealand and Fiji, and a low-grade one from New Guinea. In New Guinea especially the almost affectionate relationship between man and pigs and the ever-present contact with them, that is for reasons of attitude and ethnology, play an important role in the perpetuation of *B. suis* brucellosis in man. The exact extent of *B. suis* in man remains unknown − another, probably considerable, "grey" figure.

B. ovis, first reported in Australia in 1942 by Gunn et al. and Buddle (1956) in New Zealand seems to be a great problem for both countries with their enormous flocks of sheep. *B. ovis* affects rams especially, and after an epididymitis

Table 14. Brucellosis incidence in Australia and Oceania. (Period 1968–1975)

Country	Human cases per 100,000 Pop. p.a.	Cattle		Sheep		Goat	Swine	Game and other domestic animals
		B. ab.	B. ab.	B. mel.	B. ovis	B. mel.	B. suis	
Australia	0.97 ++	++	–	–	+	–	+	–
New Zealand	2.51 ++	+	–	–	++++	–	+	Horse + Red deer
New Guinea	+	+ and B. suis	–	–	–	–	++	Wild pig B. suis (+)
Figi-Islands	+?	+	...	...	(–)	–	+	–
New Hebrides	+?	+	–	–	–	–	–	–
New Caledonia	?	+	(–)	(–)	(–)	(+)	(–)	(–)
Western Samoa	...	–	–	–	–	–	–	–
French Polynesia	++++	+++	–	–	–	–	–	–

and orchitis it frequently leads to sterility in the infected animal. Not unlike the measures taken to control the *ovine melitensis* brucellosis the method of vaccination with Rev. 1 vaccine followed by the test-and-slaughter methods seems to lead rapidly to success (Worthington, van Tonder, Muelders 1972).

5 Conclusion

This geomedical investigation has shown that brucellosis occurs in 94 of the 153 countries in the world, and that the remaining countries have either already been successful in eradicating it or do not know about or report on its occurrence. In every case man functions as a "subsidiary host" in the epidemiology of this infectious disease, and is totally dependent in his risk of infection on the occurrence and distribution of the different brucella species in the animal host reservoirs.

The facts at present known permit the derivation of the *general epidemiological rule* that brucellosis, in accordance with its broad host spectrum and its worldwide distribution, must be presumed to be present on earth wherever cattle, sheep, goats, pigs or similar domestic animals are being kept by man or where their products are being processed and utilized. With the exception of some smaller islands, which have never been affected by brucellosis, this rule will be valid until brucellosis has been eradicated by active control measures and even detailed survey work is no longer able to detect it in man, domestic or wild animals.

Especially in the developed industrialised countries brucellosis is well on the way to eradication in domestic animals, and consequently to elimination of risk for man. The question of whether the survival and continuing residence of brucellae in wild animals away from domestic ones is to be assumed depends on local conditions. Undoubtedly sparsely settled areas with ample wild life offer sufficient opportunity for natural foci to continue to exist despite the eradication of the disease among domestic animals. The entering of wild life symbols ought to draw attention to this (see on the back of Map 3).

There are countries that stand out like islands from the sea of infection by brucellosis; they have never known it or have been succesful in its eradication. Many countries are engaged in measures to control the disease, others have not even started with it and, like some countries in, for example, Africa, Asia, Oceania or Central America, they can say little about the present state of either the frequency or the distribution of brucellosis.

All countries with animal husbandry have in common the fact that they continue to be threatened by brucellosis, be it from within or from without, and vigilance in preventing the fresh importation of the disease and the efforts to ensure its final extinction in all animal reservoirs for the protection of man must not be allowed to relax.

The health and veterinary authorities of all countries are obliged to publish information on the status of brucellosis infection as regularly as possible, and to supplement this with relevant medical and veterinary publications. In future medical cartographers will again be faced with the task of presenting the dynamic change in the incidence of brucellosis in new maps, and thus to support the efforts made for man's protection.

Acknowledgement

This book and the attached Brucellosis-Occurrence- and Distribution Maps are the result of a longlasting effort of many. The Author gratefully acknowledges the strong support by the Heidelberg Academy of Sciences for accepting the project and providing the means for data collection including travel allowances and printing.

He is deepley indebted first of all to Prof. Dr. W. Wundt, Mannheim, not only for inviting him for taking over the task and repeating his efforts from 25 years ago in mapping the world situation on the occurrence and distribution of brucellosis, but also for his personal attachment to the project, his scientific guidance and for the writing of the foreword.

But not the less to Prof. em. Dr. H. J. Jusatz, Geomedical Research Unit of the Heidelberg Academy of Sciences and to his co-workers especially Mrs. M. Albrecht and Mr. H. Sauer. All the merrits go to this team for the constant and tireless efforts in keeping the project going, supporting the questionnaire enterprise and transferring the table-data into colour and print of, what we hope, have become easily readible maps. Moreover I am very grateful to Prof. Jusatz for reading the manuscript, to Dr. J. A. Hellen, Newcastle upon Tyne, and Mrs. J. F. Hellen for the translation into English of most parts of it, to Mrs. A. Paproth and Mrs. H. Frank for caring for the typing and to the Springer Verlag, Heidelberg, and to Henning Wocke, Karlsruhe, for the marvellous printing job they have done. Especially the help of all collegues, scientists and officers at Institutes, Institutions on Ministries in freely contributing with their literature or libraries to the data-pool is very warmly acknowledged. Because of lack of space not all names can be given, but a few may be mentioned here, standing for the others: Dr. H. O. Königshöfer from the Animal Health Service, FAO, Rome, Dr. Hansluffka from the Health Statistics Service, WHO, Geneva, Dr. C. Garcia-Carillo from the Panam. Zoonosis Centre, WHO, Ramos Mejia, Argentina, Dr. R. Gaument from the Lab. Centr. Vet., Maison Alfort, Paris, Dr. W. J. Brinley Morgan, World Bruc. Reference Centre, Central Vet. Lab., Weybridge, England, Dr. T. N. Mathur, Radha Soami Satsang Beas, India; not to forget Prof. Dr. J. Boch, Institutes for Tropical Medicine, University Munich, Prof. Dr. A. Mayr, Institute for Microbiology and Infectious Diseases of Animals, Munich, and especially my friend Prof. Dr. E. Vanek, Section for Infectious Diseases, Ulm University Clinics for his constant moral support and last but not least my dear wife and children for their great patience with me during the time working on the project.

6 References

Brucellosis, General

Abdussalam M, Fein DA (1976) Brucellosis as a world problem. Internat. Symposium on Brucellosis (II) Rabat 1975. Develop biol Standard 31:9–23. Karger, Basel

Alberg SS (1973) Immunity to brucella infection. Medicine 52:339–356

Alton GG (1973) Brucellosis in goats and sheep. World Animal Rev 5:16–20

Alton GG, Jones LM, Pietz DE (1975) Laboratory techniques in brucellosis. 2nd ed Wld Hlth Org Monograph Ser No 55. WHO, Geneva

Animal health yearbooks 1954–1975. FAO, Rome

Boron P, Jezyna C, Sokolewicz-Bobrowska E, Korenkiewicz I (1975) Untersuchungen der Immunglobuline IgG, IgA und IgM im Vergleich zu immunserologischen Reaktionen bei der menschlichen, chronischen Brucellose. Z Immunitätsforsch 150:95–104

Christie AB (1969) Infectious diseases: Epidemiology and clinical practice. Livingstone Ltd, Edinburgh

Coghlan JD, Weir DM (1967) Antibodies in human brucellosis. Br Med J 2:269–271

Davidson I, Herbert CN (1978) International Standard for Anti-Brucella abortus Serum: comparison of the complement-fixing activity of the first and second International Standards and the EEC standard. Bull WHO 56:123–127

Farrell ID, Robertson L, Hinschliffe PM (1975) Serum antibody response in acute brucellosis J Hyg (Camb) 74:23–33

Hahn H (1974) Zelluläre antibakterielle Immunität. Zbl Bakt Hyg, I. Abt. Orig A 227: 184–195

Henderson RJ (1973) Brucellosis. Br J Hosp Med Nov 1973, 573–577

Henderson RJ, Hill DM, Vickers AA, Edwards JMB, Tillett HE (1975) Brucellosis and veterinary surgeons. Br Med J 2:656–659

Jones LM, Berman DT (1976) The role of living vaccines in prophylaxis. Internat Symp on Brucellosis (II), Rabat 1975. Develop biol Standard vol 31, S. Karger, Basel, pp 328–334

Kaplan MM, Abdussalam M, Biljenga G (1962) Diseases transmitted through milk. Wld Hlth Org Monograph Series No 48, Genf, pp 11–74

Kaplan MM (1969) Economic and social aspects of animal diseases in developing countries. Biotechn. Kioeng: Symposium, Genf 1:211–234

Keppie J (1964) Host and tissue specifity. Symp Soc gen Microbiol 14:44–63

Kerr WR, Coghlan JD, Payne DJH, Robertson L (1966) Chronic brucellosis in the practising veterinary surgeon. Vet Rec 79/21:602–608

Kerr WR, McCaughey WJ, Coghlan JD, Payne DJH, Quaife RA, Robertson L, Farell ID (1968) Techniques and interpretations in the serological diagnosis of brucellosis in man. J Med Microbiol 1:181–193

Krüger W (1971) Zooanthroponosen als Infektionskrankheiten. In: E Töppich (Hrsg) Leitfaden der Zooanthroponosen. VEB Verlag Volk und Gesundheit, Berlin

Lowrie DB, Kennedy JF (1972) Erythritol and threitol in canine placenta: possible implication in canine brucellosis. Febs. Letters 23:69–72

Luchsinger DW (1973) The utilitation of Brucella abortus Culturing and Biotyping Results in the Epizootiologic Investigation of Bovine Brucellosis. US Anim Health Assoc 85–99

McCullough NB (1970) Microbial and host factors in the pathogenesis of brucellosis. In: Mudd E (ed) Infectious agents and host reactions. Saunders, London, pp 324–345

McDevitt DG (1973) Symptomatology of chronic brucellosis. Brit J Ind Med 30:385–389

Morgan WJB, Gower WJ (1966) Techniques in the identification and classification of Brucella. In: Identification Methods for microbiologists, ed. Gibbs BM, Skinner FA, Academic Press, London

N N (1962) The economic losses caused by animal diseases. In: FAO Animal Health Yearbook, Geneva, pp 284–313

Parnas J, Krüger W (1966) Geoepidemiologie. In: Parnas J, Krüger W, Töppich E (Hrsg) Die Brucellose des Menschen. VEB Verlag Volk und Gesundheit, Berlin

Parnas J (1973) Die moderne Diagnostik der menschlichen Brucellose. Triangel 11:137–144

Rodenwaldt E, Jusatz HJ (Hrsg) (1952–1961) Welt-Seuchen-Atlas – World Atlas of Epidemic Diseases. Vol 1–3, Falk-Verlag, Hamburg

Roux J (1979) Epidemiology and Prevention of Brucellosis. Bull WHO 57/2:179–194

Remenzowa MM (1966) Naturherdreservoire. In: Parnas J, Krüger W, Töppich E (Hrsg) Brucellose des Menschen. VEB Verlag Volk und Gesundheit, Berlin

Scheibner E (1976) Bundesgesundheitsamt, pers. Mitteilung

Schreyer P, Caspi E, Leibe Y, Eshchar Y, Sompolinsky D (1980) Brucellosis septicaemia in pregnancy. Europ J Obstet Gynec reprod Biol 10/2:99–107

Spink WW (1975) Brucellosis. In: Wintrope MM (ed) Harrison's principles of internat medicine. 7th ed. McGraw-Hill Book Co, New York

Weber A (1979) Gegenwärtige Kenntnisse über Epidemiologie, Klinik und Diagnose der Brucellosen. Med Welt Bd 30, H 22

WHO (1971) Joint FAO/WHO Expert Committee on Brucellosis, 5th Report. Wld Hlth Org Techn Rep Ser No 464. WHO, Geneva

WHO (1972) World health statistics annual, Vol II. Infectious diseases: Cases, death and vaccinations 1968, 1969, 1970, 1971, 1972. WHO, Geneva

WHO (1972) Statistical principles in public health field studies. Wld Hlth Org techn Rep Ser No 510. WHO, Geneva

WHO (1972) Brucellosis incidence reports. WHO Statistical Report 1968–1972. WHO, Geneva

WHO (1975) World health situation, 5th Report: 1969–1972. Official Rec Wld Hlth Org No 225. WHO, Geneva

Wundt W (1961) Die Verbreitung der Brucellose auf der Erde (1930–1957), Teil III/11–16: Karte 83; – Brucellose in Europa 1929–1955, III/7–10, Karte 82. In: Rodenwaldt E, Jusatz HJ (eds) Welt-Seuchen-Atlas – World Atlas of Epidemic Diseases vol I–III, Falk Verlag Hamburg (1952–1961)

Wundt W (1978) Die Gattung Brucella-Brucellosen. In: Otte HJ, Brandis H (Hrsg) Lehrbuch der Medizinischen Mikrobiologie. G. Fischer, Stuttgart

Brucellosis in Europe and the Mediterranean Countries

Allwright SP, Murphy DL (1980) Brucellosis in Irish Meatworkers. Ir Med J 72/12:516–521

Alton GG (1969) Report to the Government of Malta on Control of Animal Brucellosis. UNDP Rep No TA 2612, FAO, Rome

Alton GG (1971) Report to the Government of Malta, Control of Animal Brucellosis. UNDP Rep No TA 2966, FAO, Rome

Alton GG (1971) Report to the Government of Cyprus, Control of Animal Brucellosis. FAO No TA 3026, 1971, Rome

Andre-Fontaine A (1980) Situation epidemiologique de la brucellose en France en 1979. Bulletin d'Information de la Chaire de Maladies Contagieuses. Ecole Nat Vet d'Alfort

Anusz Z (1978) Choroby Odzwierzece. Przeg Epid 32/1:123–127

Anusz Z (1979) Choroby Odzwierzece. Przeg Epid 33/1:153–160

Anusz Z (1980) Bruceloza I Inne Choroby Odzwierzece. Przeg Epid 34/1:111–117

Bolletino della Epizootie, Ministero della Sanita, Rep Italiana (1969–1972)

Bulgaria (1968) La Situation sanitaire et les methodes de prophylaxie appliquees en Bulgarie. Bull Off int Epiz 70:381–384

CDC (1976) Brucellosis in Swine in the Federal Republic of Germany. Vet Pub Hlth Notes 1976

Denny HR (1974) A review of brucellosis in the horse. Equine Vet J 5/3:I–V

Di Stanislao F, Renga G (1977) L'endemia Brucellare Nelle Marche. Nuovi Ann Ig Microbiol 28/6:407–427

Dziubek Z (1980) Patogeneza Zaburzen Funkcji Plciowych u Mezczyzn z Przewlekla Brucelaoza. Przeg Epid 34/1:1–9

France. Ministere de la Sante (1977) Brucellosis Surveillance. Bulletin hebdomadaire d'information epidemiologique 14. Cit. in: Wkly Epidem Rec 31:258

German Federal Republic (1971) La situation epizootique et les mesures de lutte contre les epizooties dans la Republique Federale d'Allemagne. Bull Off int Epiz 76:387–397

Golstein-Brouwers van GWM (1975) Brucella suits infecties. Tijdschr Diergeneesk 100/15:838–839

Grand-Duche de Luxembourg (1967) Bull Off int Epiz 68:339–342

Greece (1971) Brucellose. Bull Off int Epiz 76:419–425

Greus PC (1973) Estudio epidemiologico de la brucelosis en Valencia (1968–1972). Rev San Hig Pub 47:685–716

Güthenke D, Kokles R (1972) Serologische Untersuchungen an Hasenblutproben auf Leptospirose-, Brucellose-, Aujetzky- und Mucosal- Disease Antikörper. Monatsh Vet Med 27/12:465–468

Karvounaris PA (1976) Aspects cliniques et epizootioligiques de la brucellose bovine, caprine et ovine, en Grece. Develop biol Standards. Internat. Symposium on Brucellosis (II) Rabat 1975. Develop biol Standard 31:254–264. Karger, Basel

McDiarmid A (1969) Diseases in free-living wild animals. Symp. Zool Society London, Academic Press

Morgan WJB (1974) The diagnosis, control and eradication of bovine brucellosis in Great Britain. Vet Rec 94:510–517

Morgan WJB (1977) Brucellosis in Britain. Ann Sclavo 19/1:35–44

Nicolet J, Schmid Hr, Studer H, Dauwalder M (1979) Ein Ausbruch von Brucella-Suis-Biotyp-2-Infektion beim Schwein. Schweiz Arch Tierheilkd 121/5:231–238

Navarro JFM (1974) Estudio epidemiologico de la brucelosis en la provincia de Avila. Rev San Hig Pub 48:885–906

Neagle G (1980) Brucellosis in Ireland-What is Happening? Ir Med J 72/12:496–497

Off Int Epizoot, Paris (1968–1972) Animal brucellosis incidence reports of all member countries

Picheral H (1976) Espace et Sante. Geographie medicale du Midi de la France, Montpellier 133–150

Poole PM (1975) A 6-year survey of human brucellosis in a rural area of north-western England and north Wales. Postgard Med J 51:433–440

Polydorou K (1979) Brucellosis in sheep and goats in Cyprus. Com Immun Microbiol infect Dis 2:99–106

Renoux G, Renoux M (1979) Hemagglutination Passive Appliquee Au Diagnostic Individuel Ou Epidemiologique De La Brucellose Humaine. Sem Hop Paris 54/43–44:1337–1342

Rivera Perez L, Ortiz de Saracho Y Sueiro L, Quiles Pastor M (1980) Brucelosis en el Hospital Provincial de Alicante. Revision de 90 Casos. Rev Clin Esp 153/2:97–102

Roux J (1979) Surveillance des Brucelloses Humaines en France. Rev Epidemiol Sante Publique 25/5–6:427–436

Scheibner E (1974) Evolution de la brucellose porcine et lutte contre cette maladie dans la Republique Federale d'Allemagne. Bull Off int Epiz 82:113–121

Spain (1967) Prevalence de la Brucellose dans l'Espagne. Ann Rep 1967 to the FAO, Rome

Stougaard E (1974) Porcine Brucellosis in Denmark - A survey. Veterinary Services, Kopenhagen – pers. communication

Sykora I, Holda J, Sebek Z, Komarek J (1977) Eradikace Brucelozy v Chovu Psu Plemene Beagle. Vet Med 22/6:363–366

Taylor DJ (1980) Serological evidence for the presence of Brucella canis infection in dogs in Britain. Veterinary Record 106:102–103

Töppich E, Krüger W (1971) Brucellose. In: Töppich E, Krüger W (Hrsg) Leitfaden der Zooanthroponosen. VEB Verlag Volk und Gesundheit, Berlin

UdSSR (1973) Brucellosis. WHO Wkly epidem Rec 31:307

UdSSR (1973) Les Brucelloses Animales. Bull Off int Epiz 79:384

Vassiliadis P (1968) Les Brucelloses en Grèce. École d'Hygiene d'Athenes. – pers. communication

Verger JM (1973) Souches de Brucella types en 1972/73 a la Station de Pathologie de la Reproduction, INRA-Nouzilly, France – pers. communication

Wilesmith JW (1978) The persistence of Brucella abortus infection in calves: A retrospective study of heavily infected herds. Vet Rec 103:149–153

Yugoslavia (1966) Tuberculose et Brucellose Bovine. Bull Off int Epiz 66:501–515

Zourbas J, Masse L, Roussey A, David C, Maurin J, Torte J (1977) Sampling Survey on Brucellosis among Farmers and their Families in Ille-et-Vilaine (Brittany). Int J Epidemiol 6:335–343

Brucellosis in Africa

Alausa OK (1979) The investigation and control of a large-scale community outbreak of Brucellosis in Nigeria. Pub Hlth Lond 93:185–193

Alausa OK (1980) Incidence and seasonal prevalence among an occupationally-exposed population to brucellosis. Trop Gregor Med 32(1):12–15

Banerjee AK, Bhatty MA (1970) A survey of bovine brucellosis in Northern Nigeria (a preliminary communication). Bull Epizoot Dis Afr 18:333–338

Beaupere M (1966) Epizootiologie des brucelloses en Afrique noire francophone. Thesis, Ecole Nat Vet, d'Alfort, No 44

Beinhauer W (1964) Medicine veterinaire mobile. Bull Epizoot Dis Afr 12:351

Bell LM, Hayles LB, Chanda AB (1976) Evidence of reservoir hosts of brucella melitensis. Med J Zambia 10(6):152–153

Benelmouffok A (1970) Apercu sur la situation actuelle de la brucellose bovine en Algerie (Survey of the present situation of bovine brucellosis in Algeria). Arch Inst Pasteur Alger 48:207–209

Böhnel H (1971) Recherches sur les causes de mortalite des veaux dans la Savane Sous-Soudanienne du le Nord de la Cote d'Ivoire. Bull epizoot Dis Afr 19:143–157

Bouatra M (1970) Contribution a l'etude de la brucellose. Epidemiologie et prophylaxie au Maroc. These No 89, Ecole Nat Vet, Toulouse

Chambron J (1965) La brucellose bovine au Senegal. Rev Elev Med Vet Pays Trop 18:19–38

Cameron RDA, Carles AB, Lauermann Jr. LH (1971) The incidence of Brucella ovis in some Kenya flocks and its relationship to clinical lesions and semen quality. Vet Rec 89:552–556

Chantal J, Thomas JF (1976) Etude serologique sur la brucellose bovine aux abattoirs de Dakar (Serologic study of bovine brucellosis in Dakar Slaughterhouses). Rev Elev Med Vet Pays Trop 29:101–108

Collard P (1962) Antibodies against brucellae in the sera of healthy persons in various parts of Nigeria. West Afr med J 12:172

Condy JB, Vickers DB (1972) Brucellosis in Rhodesian wildlife. J S Afr Vet Med Ass 43:175–179

Cox PSV (1966) Brucellosis – a survey in South Karamoja. East Afr Med J 43:43–50

Cox PSV (1972) Human brucellosis in Kenya. Specialist Committee on Brucellosis and Tuberculosis, Muguga/Kenya 17th April, 1972

Cramlet SH, Berhanu G (1979) The relationship of Brucella abortus titers to equine fistulous withers in Ethiopia. VM SAC 74/2:195–199

Dafaala EN, Khan AQ (1958) The occurrence, epidemiology and control of animal brucellosis in the Sudan. Bull epizoot Dis Afr 6:243–247

Domenech J (1978) Serological Survey of Brucelosis of the Dromedary in Ethiopia. (Enquete serologique sur la brucellose du dromadaire en Ethiopie). Rev Elev Med Vet Pays Trop 30/2:141–142

Doutre MP, Fensterbank R, Sagna F (1977) Etude de la brucellose bovine dans un village de Basse-Casamance (Senegal). Rev Elev Med Vet Pays Trop 30/4:345–351

Essoungou NS (1970) Les brucellosis au Cameroun. Thesis, Faculte de Medicine, Lyon

Esuruoso GO, van Blake HE (1972) Bovine brucellosis in two southern states of Nigeria. An investigation of selected herds. Bull epizoot Dis Afr 20:269–274

Esuruoso GO (1974) Bovine brucellosis in Nigeria. Vet Rec 95:54–58

Eze EN (1979) Isolation of Brucellae from the Nigerian Livestock and the typing of such isolates. Bull Anim Hlth Prod Afr 26/1 29–36

Fassi-Fehri M (1975) Evolution et facteurs de diffusion de la brucellose au Maroc (Development and factors of spreading of brucellosis in Morocco). Maroc Med 55:28–32

Fensterbank R, Doutre MP, Sagna F (1977) Etude de la brucellose bovine dans un village de Basse-Casamance (Senegal). Rev Elev Med Vet Pays Trop 30/4:353–358

Fernny J, Chantal J (1976) Aspects cliniques et epidemiologiques de la brucellose bovine en Afrique tropicale (Clinical and epidemiological aspects of bovine brucellosis in tropical Africa). Dev Biol Stand 31:274–278

Food and Agriculture Organization of the United Nations (FAO) (1967) East African livestock survey, regional – Kenya, Tanzania, Uganda. Vol. I and II, Roma

Gidel R et al (1972) Resultats d'une enquete sur la brucellose humaine et animale das la region de Niamey, Rep du Niger. OCCGE-Centre Muraz, Lab Biol Sous Sect Zoonoses, No 116 – Janiver 1972

Gidel R et al (1972) Resultats d'une enquete sur la brucellose humaine et animale dans la region de Banfora, Rep de Haute-Volta. OCCGE-Centre Muraz, Lab Biol Sous Sect Zoonoses. No 71/doc du 5. 7. 1972

Gidel R, Athawet B (1975) Enquete serologique sur la brucellose humaine et les rickettsioses dans un groupe de population nomade des Regions Saheliennes de Haute-Volta (Serological survey of human brucellosis and rickettsial diseases in a group of a nomad population in the Sahelian Regions of Upper Volta). Ann Soc Belg Med Trop 55:77–83

Gidel R, Albert JP, Le Mao G, Retif M (1975) Aspects Epidemiologiques de la brucellose humaine en Afrique occidentale. Resultats de dix enquetes effectuees en Cote d'Ivoire, Haute-Vala et Niger (Epidemiological Aspects of Human brucellosis in Western Africa. Results of Surveys made in Ivory Coast, Upper Volta and Niger). Ann Soc Belg Med Trop 55:65–76

Gidel R, Albert JP, Le Mao G, Retif M (1976) Epidemiologie de la brucellose humaine et animale en Afrique de l'Quest. Develop biol Standard 31:187–200. S Karger, Basel

Gradwell DV, Schutte AP, Van Niekerk CA, Roux DJ (1977) The isolation of brucella abortus biotype 1 from African Buffalo in the Kruger National Park. J S Afr Vet Assoc 48:41–43

Guilbride, PDL et al (1962) Brucella agglutinins in the Uganda hippopotamus (Hippopotamus amphibius). J comp Path 72:137

Ghana Min Health Ann Rep. In: Epid Rep (1966) WHO, Geneva

Hoffmann H, El-Sawah HM (1969) Bovine brucellosis in the Western Zone of Tanzania. Bull epizoot Dis Afr 17:393–394

Hummel PH, Staak C (1964) Brucella abortus Biotype 3 in Tanzania. Vet Rec 94:579

Hussein AS, Singh SS, Haji H (1979) A Survey of Bovine Brucellosis in the Southern Parts of Somalia Democratic Republic. A Comparative Study of Prevalence of the Disease in Farm Animals and Animals from Nomadic Herds. Bull Anim Health Prod Afr 26/2: 150–153

Ibrahim AE, Habiballa N (1975) A survey of brucellosis in Messeriya cows of Sudan. Trop Anim Health Prod 7 (4):245–246

Kagumba M, Nandokha E (1979) A survey of the prevalence of Bovine Brucellosis in East Africa. Bull Anim Hlth Prod Afr 26/3:224–229

Klastrup NO, Halliwell RW (1977) Infectious Causes of Infertility/Abortion of Cattle in Malawi. Nord Vet Med 29:325–330

Kramer JW et al (1967) Serological survey of diseases of cattle, sheep and goats in the Eastern Provinces of Nigeria. Bull epizoot Dis Afr 15:25–29

Lasnami K (1970) Epidemiologie des brucelloses animales en Algerie. These. Lyon, Ecole Nat Vet

Mantovani A, Osman HS, Hussen AS, Nur AH, Baldelli R, Batelli G, Sanguinetti V (1975) Indagini orientative sulla presenza di brucellosi bovina nella Republica Democratica Somalia (Preliminary studies on the incidence of bovine brucellosis in the Democratic Republic of Somalia). Ann Sclavo 17:179–180

Manson-Bahr PEC (1956) Clinical aspects of brucellosis in East Africa. East Afr Med J 33:489–494

Mansvelt PR (1975) Brucellosis in the Republic of South Africa (pers. communication)

Mauretania: Bovine brucellosis: Vet Dept Rep (1971) Bull Off int Epiz 76:483–487

Mortelmans J, Kageruka P (1970) A propos de la brucellose et des souches de brucella en Afrique Centrale. Int Symp on Brucellosis, Tunis 1968. Symp Ser Immunobiol Standard 12:207–210. Karger, Basel

Nagy LK, Sorheim AO (1969) A survey of brucella infection of cattle in Kenya. Vet Rec 84:65–67

Ndyabahinduka DG (1980) Brucellosis: An increasing public health hazard in Uganda. Ann Ist Super Sanita 14/2:229–234

Newton FJ, Jones E, Connor RJ, Davidson BJ, McGovern PT (1974) A survey of bovine brucellosis in four districts of Uganda. Br Vet J 130:249–254

Okoh AEJ, Alexiev I, Agbonlahor DE (1978) Brucellosis in Dogs in Kano, Nigeria. Trop Anim Hlth Prod 10:219–220

Omer EE, Habiballa N, Dafaalla EA (1978) Evaluation of the Standard Agglutination Test in the Diagnosis of Human Brucellosis in the Sudan. J Trop Med Hyg 81/10:190–194

Oomen LJA, Wegener J (1974) Brucellosis. In: Vogel LC et al (eds) Health and Disease in Kenya. East African Literature Bureau, Nairobi, pp 221–224

Oomen LJA (1976) Human brucellosis in Kenya. Trop geogr Med 28:45–53

Opitz HM (1969) Brucellosis in Sierra Leone, a serological survey in cattle, sheep and goats. Bull Epizoot Dis Afr 17:383–391

Opong ENW (1966) Bovine brucellosis in Southern Ghana. Bull Epizoot Dis Afr 14:397–403

Philpott M, Auko O (1972) Caprine brucellosis in Kenya. Brit Vet J 128:642–651

Plagemann O (1974) Ein Beitrag zur Rinderbrucellose in Uganda (Bovine brucellosis in Uganda). Berl Münch Tierärztl Wochenschr 87:173–175

Richard C (1966) Les brucelloses animales au Senegal. Thesis, Ecole Nat Vet d'Alfort, No 43

Rollinson DHL (1962) Brucella agglutinins in East African game animals. Vet Rec 74:904

Roux J, Baylet R (1971) Quelques donnees sur l'epidemiologie des Brucelloses au Senegal. Med Afr Noire 18:813–815

Sachs R, Staak C, Groocock CM (1968) Serological investigation of brucellosis in game animals in Tanzania. Bull Epizoot Dis Afr 16:93–100

Sacquet E (1955) La brucellose bovine au Tchad. Rev Elev Med Vet Pays Trop 8:5–7

Schiemann P, Staak C (1971) Brucella melitensis in Impala (Aepyceros melampus). Vet Rec 88:344

Staak C, Groocock C, Sachs R (1967) Brucellose-Untersuchungen auf Farmen im Massailand und beim Wild im nördlichen Gebiet von Tanzania. Berl Münch Tierärztl Wochenschr 80:8–11

Staak C (1972) Brucellosis reservoir in almost uncontrolable areas. Specialist Committee on brucellosis and tuberculosis. East African Veterinary Research Organization. Meeting 17th April, 1972, Muguga/Kenya

Staak C, Protz D (1973) A brucellosis survey in the Massailand and Mbulu District of Tanzania. Bull Epizoot Dis Afr 21:67–74

Schutte AP (1978) Brucellose in Suid-Afrika en die Rol van die Veearts. J S Afr Vet Assoc 48/3:177–181

Thienpont D et al (1958) Recherches sur la brucellose bovine et humaine au Congo Belge et au Ruanda-Urundi, a propos d'une enquete dans le territoire d'Astrida (R-U). Ann Soc Belg Med Trop 38:1049–1073

Thimm B (1971) Zoonosen und ihre Bedeutung für die Entwicklung der tierischen Produktion in Ostafrika II. Das Beispiel Brucellose. Schlacht- und Viehhof Zeitung 5:178–185

Thimm B (1972) Brucellosis in Uganda. Part I: The epizootiological and epidemiological situation. Bull Epizoot Dis Afr 20:43–56

Thimm B (1973) Zum Problem einer erhöhten angeborenen Resistenz der ostafrikanischen Kurzhorn-Zeburasse (Bos indicus) gegenüber Brucellose. Zbl Vet Med B 20:490–494

Thimm B, Nauwerck G (1974) Bovine brucellosis in Guinea and West Africa. Zbl Vet Med B 21:692–705

Thimm B, Wundt W (1976) The epidemiological situation of brucellosis in Africa. Internat. Symposium on Brucellosis (II), Rabat 1975. Develop biol Standard 31:201–217. Karger, Basel

Thimm B, Wundt W (1976) Methode der monographischen Bearbeitung der globalen Verbreitung einer Krankheit. Dargestellt am Beispiel der Brucellose bei Mensch und Tier. In: Jusatz JG (Hrsg) Methoden und Modelle der geomedizinischen Forschung. Erdkundliches Wissen Heft 43. Franz Steiner, Wiesbaden, S 32–35

Vacic L (1972) La brucellose bovine et procine en Republique Populaire du Congo. Rapport d'Avancement No 2, p 9 (15. 1. 1972). AGA Project COB-69/4. FAO, Rome

Vanek E (1976) Epidemiologisch-serologische Untersuchungen über die Brucellose und das Q-Fieber in Kenia/Ostafrika. Habilitationsschrift Univ Ulm

Verger JM, Gate M, Piechaud M, Chatelain R, Ramisse J, Blancou J (1975) Isolement de Brucella suis biotype 5a Madagaskar, chez une chienne, validite du nom d'espece Brucella canis. Ann Microbiol (Paris) 126:57–74

Verger JM, Grayon M, Doutre MP, Sagna F (1979) Brucella abortus d'origine bovine au Senegal: identification et typage. Rev Elev Med Vet Pays Trop 32/1:25–32

Waghela S, Fazil MA, Gathuma JM, Kagunya DK (1978) A serological survey of Brucellosis in Camels in North-Eastern Province of Kenya. Trop Anim Hlth Prod 10/1:28–29

Waghela S (1979) Animal Brucellosis in Kenya: A Review. Bull Anim Hlth Prod Afr 24/1:53–59

Wernery U, Kerani AA, Viertel P (1979) Bovine Brucellosis in the Southern Regions of the Somali Democratic Republic. Trop Anim Hlth Prod 11:31–35

Worthington RW, Tonder, van EM, Muelders MS (1972) The incidence of Brucella ovis infection in South African rams: A serological survey. J S Afr Vet Assoc 43:83–85

Wright FJ, Cooke ERN, D'Souza JStAM (1953) Observations on brucellosis in Kenya. Trans R Soc Trop Med Hyg 47:117–129

Zaire, Kivu Vet Dept. Annual Report (1959)

Brucellosis in North America

Acosta M, Ludena H, Barret D, Moro M (1972) Brucelosis en Alpacas. Rev Inv Pec (IVITA) Univ Nac S Marcos 1/1:37–49

Adlam GH (1973) Brucellosis, National Disease Eradication Scheme. Bull Off int Epiz 79/5–6:447–448

Anderson RK, Berry WT, Wise R, Berman DT, Hopkin JA (1978) National Brucellosis Technical Commission Report. National Technical Information Service, Springfield, VA, USA

Barton CL (1978) Canine Brucellosis. Vet Clin North Am 7/4:705–710

Barrett MW, Chalmers GA (1975) A serologic survey of Pronghorns in Alberta and Saskatchewan, 1970–1972. J Wildl Dis 11:157–163

Becker HN, Belden RC, Brault T, Burridge MJ, Frankenberger WB, Nicoletti P (1979) Brucellosis in Feral Swine in Florida. J AM Vet Med Assoc 173/9:1181–1182

Boerr WJ, Crawford RP, Hidalgo RJ, Robinson RM (1980) Small Mammals and White-Tailed Deer as possible Reservoir Hosts of Brucella Abortus in Texas. J Wildl Dis 16/1:19–24

Brody JA, Huntley B, Overfield ThM, Maynard J (1966) Studies of Human Brucellosis in Alaska. J Inf Dis 116:263–269

Brown GM (1977) The History of the Brucellosis Eradication Program in the United States. Ann Sclavo 19/1:20–34

Broughton E, Choquette LPE, Cousineau JG, Miller FL (1970) Brucellosis in reindeer (Rangifer tarandus L.) and the migratory barren-ground caribou (Rangifer tarandus groenlandicus L.) in Canada. Can J Zool 48/5:1023–1027

Buchanan T, Faber C, Feldman R (1974) Brucellosis in the United States, 1960–1972. Medicine 53:403–413

Buchanan T, Sulzer CR, Frix MK, Feldman RA (1974) Brucellosis in the United States, 1960–1972. Medicine 53:415–425

Buchanan T, Hendricks SL, Patton CM, Feldman RA (1974) Brucellosis in the United States, 1960–1972. Medicine 53:427–439

Carmichael LE, George LW (1976) Canine brucellosis: newer knowledge. Internat. Symposium on Brucellosis (II) Rabat 1975. Develop biol Standard 31:237–250. Karger, Basel

Center for Disease Control (1979) Morbidity and Mortality Weekly Report. Brucellosis – United States, 1978. US Department of Health, Education, and Welfare 28/37:437–448

CDC (1975) Brucellosis Surveillance Annual Summary, 1974. US Dept Hlth Ed Welf, Atlanta Ga

CDC (1976) Brucellosis Eradication in the United States. Vet Pub Hlth Notes March 1976

CDC (1976, 1977) Reported Morbidity & Mortality in the United States. US Dept Hlth Ed Welfare, Publ Hlth Serv, Atlanta, Georgia

Choquette LP, Broughton E, Cousineau JG, Novakowski NS (1979) Parasites and diseases of Bison in Canada IV. Serologic Survey for Brucellosis in Bison in Northern Canada. J Wildl Dis 14/3:329–332

Crawford RP, Williams JD, Childers AB, Hidalgo RJ, Huber JD, Boyd CL (1978) The Effects of Brucella Abortus on Serology Bacteriology, and Production in three Texas Cattle Herds. Proc Ann Meet US Anim Health Assoc 82:89–105

Davis DS, Boeer WJ, Mims JP, Heck FC (1979) Brucella abortus in Coyotes. I. A serologic and bacteriologic survey in Eastern Texas. J Wildl Dis 15/3:367–372

DeLong WJ, Waldhalm DG, Hall RF (1979) Bacterial Isolates Associated with Epididymitis in Rams from Idaho and Eastern Oregon Flocks. Am J Vet Res 40/1:101–102

Drazek FJ (1978) Bovine Disease Control Problems in the Northeast. IB. Brucellosis-Current Status. Cornell Vet 68/7:173–178

Gray MD, Martin SW (1980) An Evaluation of Screening Programs for the Detection of Brucellosis in Dairy Herds. Can J Comp Med 44/1:52–60

Hampy B, Pence DB, Simpson CD (1980) Serological Studies on Sympatric Barbary Sheep and Mule Deer from Palo Duro Canyon, Texas. J Wildl Dis 15/3:443–446

Hoff GL, Schneider NJ (1975) Serologic survey for agglutinins to Brucella canis in Florida residents. Amer J Trop Med Hyg 24:157–159

Hudson M, Child KN, Hatler DF, Fujino KK, Hodson KA (1980) Brucellosis in Moose. A Serological Survey in an Open Range Cattle Area of North Central British Columbia Recently Infected with Bovine Brucellosis. Can Vet J 21:47–49

Johnson BG (1978) Status of the Cooperative State-Federal Brucellosis Eradication Program. Proc Ann Meet US Anim Health Assoc 82:157–172

Kien L, Deckelbaum R, Mishkin S, Wiglesworth FW, Brazeau M (1974) Brucellosis in the Eskimo Child. Can J Pub Hlth 65:202–203

Kooy P (1970) Brucellosis, Treponematosis, Rickettsiosis, and Psittacosis in Surinam. A serological Survey. Trop geogr Med 22:172–178

Kourany DM, Vasquez RMM (1975) Encuesta Seroepidemiologica de Brucelosis en una Poblacion de Alto Reisgo en Panama. Bol Of Sanit Panam 79:230–236

Malkin KL, Tailyour JM, Bhatia TRS, Archibald RMcG, Dorward WJ (1968) A serological survey for Brucellosis in Canadian Swine. Can J comp Med 32:598–599

Martin SW, Gerrow AF (1978) The use of case history studies to differentiate potentially infected from potentially noninfected herds with reactors to Brucella abortus antigen. Can J comp Med 42/1:16–22

Merell CL, Wright DN (1978) A serologic survey of Mule Deer and Elk in Utah. J Wildl Dis 14/4:471–478

Monroe PW, Silberg SL, Morgan PM, Adess M (1975) Seroepidemiological investigation of Brucella canis antibodies in different human population groups. J Clin Microbiol 2:382–386

Nadler HE (1978) Bovine Disease Control Problems in the Northeast. IA. Brucellosis: An Overview. Cornell Vet 68/7:164–172

Neiland KA (1970) Rangiferine Brucellosis in Alaskan Canids. J Wildl Dis 6:136–139

Neiland KA (1975) Further observations on Rangiferine Brucelllosis in Alaskan carnivores. J Wildl Dis 11/1:45–53

Nelson KE, Ruben FL, Andersen B (1978) An Unusual Outbreak of Brucellosis. Arch Intern Med 135/5:691–695

Ossola AL, Szyfres B, Blood B (1963) Natural Infection of sheep by Brucella melitensis in Argentina. Am J Vet Res 24/100:446–449

Pan American Sanitary Bureau, Reg Off Wld Hlth Org (1974) Pan American Zoonoses Center Regional Project. Semi-Annual Report. Washington

Pickerill PA, Carmichael LE (1972) Canine Brucellosis: Control Programs in Commercial Kennels and Effect on Reproduction. J Amer Vet Med Ass 160/12:1607–1615

Snell E (1964) Brucellosis in Manitoba. Can J Pub Hlth 55:247–250

Stauber EH, Authenrieth R, Markman OD, Whitbeck V (1980) A seroepidemiologic survey of three Pronghorn (Antilocapra americana) populations in southeastern Idaho, 1975–1977
Thorne ET, Morton JK, Thomas GM (1978) Brucellosis in Elk. I. Serologic and Bacteriologic Survey in Wyoming. J Wildl Dis 14/1:74–81
Toshach S (1963) Brucellosis in the Canadian Arctic. Can J Pub Hlth 54:271–275
Vaughn HW, Knight RR, Frank FW (1973) A study of reproduction, disease and physiological blood and serum values in Idaho Elk. J Wildl Dis 9:296–300

Brucellosis in South- and Central America and the Caribic

Agosta M, Ludena H, Barreto D, Moro M (1972) Brucelosis en Alpacas. Rev Inv Pec (IVITA) Univ Nac S Marcos 1:37–49
Amechino EC, Veliz QFN (1970) Epidemiologia de la Brucelosis Ovina en la Sierra Central. Cuarto Boletin extraordinario, Inst Vet Invest Trop Alt (IVITA), Lima, Peru, pp 268–282
Argentina. Secretaria de Estado de Agricultura y Ganaderia de la Nation, Servicio National de Sanidad Animal (1977) Brucelosis. Servicio de Luchas (SELSA). Epizootiological Bulletin. Buenos Aires
Bahamas. Ministerio de Agricultura (1974) Status of certain zoonoses in the Americas, according to condition of the disease and control programs. Annual Zoonoses Report to the Panamerican Zoonosis Centre of the WHO, Ramos Mejia, Argentina
Barbados. Ministerio de Agricultura (1974) Status of certain zoonoses in the Americas, according to condition of the disease and control programs. Annual Zoonosis Report to the Panamerican Zoonosis Centre of the WHO, Ramos Mejia, Argentina
Barg L, Godoy AM, Peres JN (1977) Pequisa de aglutininas anti-Brucella canis em soros humanos. Arq Esc Vet UFMG 29/1:31–34
Baruffa G (1978) Prevalencia sorologica da Brucelose na zona sul do Rio Grande Do Sul (Brasil). Rev Inst Med trop Sao Paulo 20/2:71–75
Bavera GA (1971) La Infeccion Brucelica en 6253 Vacunos correspondientes a 105 Tambos de la Cuenca Lechera de Coronel Moldes – Cordoba. Rev Med Vet 52/4:319–327
Belize. Ministerio de Agricultura (1975) Country report to the VIII Reunion Interamericana (RICAZ) Meeting
Bolivia. Ministerio de Asuntos Campesinos y Agropecuarios (1974) Programa Nacional de control de la Fiebre Aftosa, Rabia y Brucelosis
Brasil. Ministerio de Agricultura (1976). Campanhas Sanitarias. Informe combate a Brucelose Animal
Brasil. Ministerio de Agricultura (1977) Diagnostico de Saude Animal. Programa Nacional de Saude Animal. Brasilia
Carpio M, Patino D, Gonzales S (1973) Estudio sobre Brucelosis en Bovinos de carne del area de Pucallpa. Rev Inv Pec (IVITA) Univ Nac S Marcos 2/1:113–114
Castagnino D, Regelado P (1970) Brucelosis Bovina en Piura, I+II. Su Incidencia en un Rebano de carne. Cuarto Boletin éxtraordinario, Inst Vet Invest Trop Alt (IVITA), Lima, Peru, pp 210–212, 213–214
Cattebeke R, Pedretti J, Dickey J (1974) Determinacion de la incidencia de la brucelosis en el ganado bovino de carne en el Paraguay. Proniega, Informe Annual 1974
Cedro VCF (1968) Swine Brucellosis Prophylaxis in Argentina. WHO/FAO Inter-Regional Seminar on Brucellosis. Pendik, Istanbul 16–27 April 1968
Cedro VCF (1968) Report on Brucellosis in Argentina. WHO/FAO Inter-Regional Seminar on Brucellosis, Pendik, Istanbul 16–27 April 1968
Centro Panamericano de Zoonosis (1974, 1975, 1977, 1978) Brucelllosis. Boletin Informativo. Ramos Mejia, Prov de Buenos Aires, Argentina
Chile. Servicio Agricola y Ganadero, Division de Salud Animal (1975) Resumen del Proyecto de control y erradicacion de la Brucelosis bovina. Boletin de Informacion Cientifica y Tecnica 9/Julio-Agosto pp:36–38. Santiago, Chile
Columbia. Ministerio de Agricultura (1974) Subproyecto de Sanidad, Programa Nacional de combate de la Brucelosis. Inferme Annual 1974
Costa EO de (1973) Sobre a ocorrencia de brucelose em bufalos (Bubalus bubalis) no Estado de Goias. Inquerito serologico. O Biol 39:162–164

52   References

Costa Rica. Ministerio de Agricultura y Ganaderia, San Jose (1974) Informe de la situacion zoosanitaria e el pais ano 1974. Brucelosis. Report to the VIII Reunion Interamericana sobre el control de la Fiebre Aftosa y otras zoonosis

Cuba. Havana (1967) Symposium on Zoonoses. Bol Hig Epidem 5/3:277–532. Cit in: Abstr. Hyg (1969) 44/3:179–180

Cuba. Ministerio de Agricultura (1975) Programa Nacional de Salud Animal. Brucelosis, Tuberculosis y Rabia en Bovinos

Eckman MR (1975) Brucellosis Linked to Mexican Cheese. JAMA 232:636–637

Ecuador. Ministerio de Agricultura y Ganaderia (1978) Brucellosis. Diagnostico de Brucelosis en Bovinos segun provincias Ecuador 1977. Boletin 1, Programa Nacional de Sanidad National, Quito, Ecuador

El Salvador. Ministerio de Agricultura (1975) Analysis y complementacion del diagnostico de la situacion sanitaria de la ganaderia en la Rebublica de El Salvador. Incidencia de Brucelosis Bovina 1970–1974

Escalante JA, Held JR (1969) Brucellosis in Peru. J.A.V.M.A. 155/12:2146–2152

Fernandez OO (1974) Brucellosis situation in animals in Argentina. pers. communication

Galvez OE (1969) Brucelosis en Cerdos de Abasto de la Ciudad de Guatemala. Rev Fac Med Vet y Zoot 2/3:34–35

Garcia-Carillo C, Szyfres B, Gonzales Tome J (1972) Tipificacion de brucelas aisladas del hombre y los animales en America Latina. Rev lat amer Microbiol 14:117–125

Garcia JFE (1976) Investigacion de anticuerpos contra "Brucella canis" en la especie canina en la Cuidad Capital. Thesis, Univ S Carlos Guatemala

Godoy AM, Peres JN, Barg L (1977) Isolamento de Brucella canis em Minas Gerais, Brasil. Arq Esc Vet UFMG 29/1:35–42

Grinling K (1973) Malta Fever in Peru. World Health, WHO, Sept 1973

Guatemala. Ministerio de Agricultura; Direccion de Ganaderia (1975) Programa Nacional de Medicina Preventiva. Brucelosis. Informe de Guatemala

Guyana. Ministerio de Agricultura (1974) Status of certain zoonoses in the Americas, according to condition of the disease and control programs. Report to the Panamerican Zoonosis Centre of the WHO, Ramos Mejia, Argentina

Haiti. Ministerio de Agricultura (1974) Situation de quelques zoonoses dans les Americas dápres l état de la maladie et les programmes de lutte. Report to the Panamericano Zoonosis Centre of the WHO, Ramos Mejia, Argentina

Honduras. Secretaria de Recursos Naturales (1973) Proyecto de Sanidad Animal para el control y eradicacion de Brucelosis y Tuberculosis bovina. 1:23–139; 2:1–6

Ibanez A, Nicholls MJ, King CT (1975) Prevalencia de la Brucelosis en ganado bovino de carne en la Region Oriental del Paraguay. Cit in: Paraguay. Ministerio de Agricultura y Ganadderia (1976) Programa Nacional de Salud Animal

Ibanez AA, Nicholas MJ, King CT (1977) A survey of brucellosis in beef cattle in Paraguay. Brit vet J 133:405–411

Jamaica. Ministerio de Agricultura. (1975) Brucelosis. Country Report 1974. Informe para la VIII Reunion Interamericana a Nivel Ministerial sobre Fiebre Aftosa y Otros Zoonoses, Guatemala

Lombardo RA (1971) Panorama general de la Brucellosis en las Americas. Grupo Estudo sobre Brucelosis. Washington, D.C. 17–19. 2. 1971. Centro Panamericano de Zoonosis, WHO, Ramos Mejia, Argentina

Lopez ET, Garza FLG (1970) Prevalencia de la Brucelosis Caprina en Tamaulipas, Mexico. Bol Of San Panam 69/4:237–290

Mejia B (1979) Brucelosis en personal de un matadero de caldas, Columbia. Bol Of Sanit Panam 87/4:319–324

Mendoza HM (1972) Prevalencia de Brucelosis del Ganado Bovino en el Departamento de Jinotega, Nicaragua. Thesis, Univ S Carlos, Guatemala

Mexico. Secretaria de Agricultura y Ganaderia; Direccion General de Sanidad Animal (1975) Advances de la Campana contra la Brucelosis. Informe para la VIII Reunion Interamericana a Nivel Ministerial sobre Fiebre Aftosa y Otras Zoonosis, Guatemala

Miranda LDP, Manrique GR (1975) Prevalencia de la Brucelosis Humana, en Hatos Bovinos Infectados Y en Mataderos del Departamento del Valle del Cauca. Rev Inst Colomb Agropecu 10/2:195–206

Moro MS (1970) Infeccion por Brucella ovis. Univ Nac M San Marcos, Rev Inv Pecuarias (IVITA) Cuarto Boletin Extraordinario, Lima, pp 290–295

Nicaragua. Ministerio de Agricultura (1974) Informe sobre la situacion actual de algunas zoonosis en la Rep de Nicaragua, segun la condicion de la enfermedad y los programas de lucha contre las mismas

Ogassawara S, Cury R, Dapica VP, Mendes MFM, Rocha UF (1969) Higroma articular Brucelico em Bufalo (Bubalus Bubalis, L). Arq Inst Biol 36/2:117–121

Panama. Ministerio de Agricultura (1974) Situacion de algunas zoonosis en las Americas, segun condicion de la enfermedad y programas de lucha. Report to the Centro Panamericano de Zoonosis of the WHO, Ramos Mejia, Argentina

Paraguay. Ministerio de Agricultura y Ganaderia (1976) Programa Nacional de Salud Animal. Brucelosis, Tuberculosis y Rabia en Bovinos

Peru. Ministerio de Alimentation (1974) Situacion de Algunas Zoonosis en el Peru, Informe Sumarizado; Periodo 1974, pp 1–4

Pinedo Sanchez A, Rubio Parra V, Sancho Garcia E (1978) La brucelosis en la provincia de Ciuded Real: Caracteristicas epidemiologicas y sociales (1). Rev San Hig Pub 52:919–932

Portugal MASC, Nesti A, Giorgi A, Franca FN, Oliviera B de (1971) Brucelose em equideos determinada por Brucella suis (Brucellosis among equines caused by Brucella suis). Arq Inst Biol, Sao Paulo, 38/3:125–132

Republica Dominicana. Secretaria de Estado de Agricultura. Direccion General de Ganaderia (1976) Proyecto de Reglamento para el control y la profillaxis de la Brucelosis, Tuberculosis y Garrapatosis del Ganado, Santo Domingo

Santa Rosa CA, Da Silva AS, Giorgi W, Machado A (1973) Isolamento de Leptospira, Sorotipo Pomona e Brucello suis, de Suinos do Estado de Santa Catarina. Arq Inst Biol 40/1:29–32

Soriano F, Miramontes MCP, Ales JM, Rubio PGH (1978) Anticuerpos anti-Brucella canis en diferentes grupos de poblacion. Una investigacion seroepidemiologica. Rev Cli Esp 149/3:247–250

Souza AP, Filho DM, Favero M (1977) Investigacao da brucelose em bovinos e em consumidores humanos do leite. Rev Saude publ, Sao Paulo 11:238–247

Szyfres B, Gonzales Tome J (1967) Natural brucella infection in wild foxes in Argentina. Bol Of San Panam 62:144–150

Szyfres B (1973) Situation de la brucelosis en America Latina. Report al Primer Seminario Nacional sobre Brucelosis, Caracas, Venezuela. Centro Panamericano de Zoonosis, Buenos Aires, Argentina

Turovetzky A, Lucero N, Garcia-Carillo, C (1979) Brucella abortus Biotipo 2 aislada de un Paciente en la Republica Argentina. Medicina (Buenos Aires) 39:99–100

Uruguay. Ministerio de Agricultura y Pesca, Montevideo (1976) Proyecto Sanidad Animal; Sub-Proyecto de Brucelosis. pp 98–111

Varela-Diaz VM, Myers DM (1979) Occurance of antibodies to Brucella canis in rural inhabitants of Corrientes and Neuquen Provinces, Argentina. Am J Trop Med Hyg 28/1:110–113

Vaughn JB, Newell KW, Brayton JB, Barth RAJ, Gracian M (1967) Encuesta sobre las Zoonosis en Mataderos de Colombia. Bol Of San Panam 1967/1:17–29

Venezuela. Ministerio de Agricultura y Cria, Division de Sanidad Animal (1971–1976) Brucelosis. Boletin de Enfermedades de los Animales Domesticos de Declaration Oficial Obligatoria

Vincente Martin V de, Onorbe M, Beato A, Gonzalez C (1978) Estudio epidemiologico de la brucelosis en la provincia de Guadalajara. Rev San Hig Pub 52:843–893

Zamora J, Luchsinger E, Martin R (1967) Brucelosis canina, Area rural de Valdivia (Chile). Rev lat-amer Microbiol Parasitol 9:69–71

Zapatel J, Malaga H (1971) Epidemiologia de la brucelosis caprina en el Peru. Bol Of Sanit Panam 71/2:121–131

Brucellosis in Asia, Australia and Oceania

Alton GG, Gulasekharam J (1974) Brucellosis as a human health hazard in Australia. Austr Vet J 50:209–215

Anand BR (1966) Distribution of agglutinins for enteric group of organisms, brucellae and rickettsiae in the population of the Kaschmir Valley. Indian J Med Sci 20:1–5

Arambulo PV (1974) The natural nidality of zoonoses in the Philippines. Int J Zoon 1:58–74

Australia (1973) Bovine Brucellosis. Bull Off int Epiz 79/5–6:441–444

Chitkara NL, Kaur H (1966) Serological study of brucellosis in man in Punjab. J Ind Med Ass 46:368

Chowdhury TM, Chatterjee A (1975) Preliminary serological survey of brucellosis in animal and man. Indian J Anim Health 14:83–84

Danusantoso H (1972) A review of brucellosis in Indonesia with report of a recent case. Southeast Asian J Trop Med Pub Health 3:314–318

Dennis SM (1974) Perinatal lamb mortality in Western Australia. Austr Vet J 50:507–510

Dhodapkar PG, Singh T (1971) Incidence of brucellosis in equines with special reference of abortions. J Remont Vet Corps 10/1:11

Fazli SA (1970) A serological survey on brucellosis in Aphganistan. Mikrobiyol Bult 4/3:105–110

Feiz J, Sabbaghian H, Miralai M (1979) Brucellosis due to B. melitensis in children. Clinical and epidemiologic observations on 95 patientes studied in Central Iran. Clin Pediatr (Phila) 17/12:904–907

Finau SA, Reinhardt GN (1980) Human Brucellosis in Tonga. NZ Med J 91:386–388

Gatapia SL, Castillo AM, Carlos RS (1971) A survey of the incidence of brucellosis among cattle and carabaos slaughtered at the National Abattoir. Manila, Philippines – pers. communication

Indonesia (1973) Brucellosis. Bull Off int Epiz 79/5–6:435–440

Israel (1966) Brucellosis in cattle, sheep and goats. Bull Off int Epiz 66:539–548

Japan (1973) Brucellosis. Bull Off int Epiz 79/3–4:373

Karim MA, Penjouian EK, Dessouky FI (1980) The prevalence of brucellosis among sheep and goats in Northern Iraq. Trop Anim Hlth Prod 11/3:186–188

Kikuchi YK et al (1979) A survey of Brucella canis infection in dogs sheltered in Tohoku University School of Medicine. Exp Anim 28/2:279–286

Krishna Rao C (1970) Epizootiology, diagnosis and control of brucellosis in India. Bull Off int Epizoot 73 (1–2):3–7

Mahakur RC, Panda GK (1972) Incidence of brucellosis in and around Burla. Ind J Med Sci 26:826

Mathur TN (1958) Human brucellosis in Punjab and its importance to the veterinarians. Indian vet J 36:181

Mathur TN (1.64) Brucella strains isolated from cows, bufalloes, goats, sheep and human beings at Karnal: Their significance with regard to the epidemiology of Brucellosis. Ind J Med 52/1:240–241

Mathur TN (1964a) The role of goat in human brucellosis in India with particular reference to infection with Brucella melitensis. J Ass Physicians India 12:806

Mathur TN (1967) Isolation of Brucella abortus from goats and sheep in Punjab. Indian vet Sci 37:277–286

Mathur TN (1968) A study of human brucellosis based on cultures isolated from man and animals. Indian J Med Res 56/3:250–258

Mathur TN (1969) A study of 232 cases of brucellosis in Karnal. Indian J Med Ass 53/8:386–390

McKay Anzinolt EJ (1972) Human Brucellosis in the Waikato: Some aspects concerning Laboratory Diagnosis. New Zealand Med J 76:265–269

Nanda BK, Mohanty SK, Nathsarma KC, Dasch S, Mishra SC (1979) Prevalence of brucella agglutinins in sera of patients suffering from pyrexia of unknown origin in Southern Orissa. Indian J Path Micorb 22:61–64

Nandgoankar D, Narayana Rao PL (1971) A survey of the incidence of bovine brucellosis in the integrated milk project area and in some of the dairy farms of Andhra Pradesh. Indian Vet 48/1:12–18

Nobuto K, Suto K (1970) Present situation of brucellosis in Japan. Bull Off int Epiz 73/1–2:17–27

Norton TH, Thomas AD (1976) Letter: Brucella suis in feral pigs. Austr Vet J 52:293–294

Oszan K, Fazh A, Aktan M, Beyoglu K (1976) Brucellosis, Tularaemia and Borreliosis isolated from Wild Animals captured in Ankara, Konya, Urfa and Nevsehir Provinces in Turkey. Mikrobiyol Bul 10:413–421

Panda SN (1968) Studies on animal brucellosis in Orissa. Bull Ind Soc Mal Com Dis 5/3–4:217–219

Ram T, Sharma RM, Kalra DS (1964) Incidence of brucellosis in animals in Punjab and its control. J Res (PAU) 1:158

Rhandawa AS, Dhillon SS (1974) Seroprevalence of brucellosis in humans and animals of Punjab. Ind J Pub Hlth 18/1:15–21

Sabbaghian H, Nadim H (1974) Epidemiology of human brucellosis in Isfahan, Iran. J Hyg Camb 73:221–228

Saegusa J, Ueda K, Goto Y, Fujiwara K (1978) A survey of Brucella canis Infection in dogs from Tokyo area. Jap J vet Sci 40:75–80

Serikawa T, Muraguchi T, Nakao N (1977) A survey of dogs from Gifu and Shiga area for Brucella canis. Jap J vet Sci 39:635–642

Sen R, Das M (1970) A note on brucellosis in and around Calcutta. Indian J Med Res 58:684

Sen GP, Joshi TP, Singh G (1972) Incidence of brucellosis among pigs in India – s short note. Ind Vet J 49:971–973

Sen GP, Joshi TP, Singh G (1974) Brucellosis among horses in India – A serological study. Equine Vet J 6/2:94–96

Sen GP, Sharma GL (1975) Speciation of seventy-eight Indian strains of brucella – An epidemiological study. Indian J Anim Sci 45/8:537–542

Sen GP, Khanna PN (1977) Role of Brucella and Coxiella burnetti infections in pyrexia of unknown origin. Indian J Pub Hlth 21/3:149–156

Sharma KD, Patil SD, Talib VH (1973) Survey of brucellosis at Aurangabad. Indian J Med Sci 27:546–549

Sharma VD, Sethi MS, Yadav MP (1979) Sero-epidemiologic investigations on Brucellosis in the States of Uttar Pradesh (U.P.) and Delhi (India). Int J Zoon 6:75–81

Shivdekar DS, Pathak PN (1969) Search for specific Brucella Agglutinins in goats milk. Ind Vet J 46/4:275–278

Singh B (1964) Agglutinins against brucella species in sera of healthy individuals and febrile patients. Ind J Path Bact 7:86

Sivarajan VL, Lakshmiah CS, Sakthivel GV (1965) Human brucellosis in Tanjavur. Ind J Med Sci 19:395

Sreenivasan R (1972) Incidence of brucellosis in the endemic areas of Tamilnadu. Cheiron 1:1

Subharngkasen S (1970) Brucellosis in Thailand. Bull Off int Epiz 73/1–2:9–15

Tadjebakche H, Gatel A (1972) Incidence serologique des anticorps antibrucelliques chez les animaux domestiques et l'homme en Iran. Rev Elev Med Vet Pay Trop 25/4:521–525

Turkey (1971) Bovine Brucellosis. Bull Off int Epiz 76:435–441

Ueda K et al (1974) Detection of B. canis infection on dogs in Tokyo area. Jap J vet Sci 36:539–542

Unel S (1968) Investigations on B. melitensis in cheese. UNDP/FAO Sheep Diseases Laboratories, Pendik, Turkey

Vejjajiva S, Yenbruta D, Pranich K, Pipitkul S (1970) Brucella agglutinins in the Thais. J Med Ass Thailand 53/6:407–410

Watt DA (1970) Investigations of Ovine Brucellosis in Merino Rams of Western Australia. Austr Vet J 46:506–508

Yamauchi C et al (1974) Canine Brucellosis in a Beagle Breeding Colony. Jap J vet Sci 36:175–182

Young JS, Blair JM (1974) Perinatal lamb losses in beef herds. Austr Vet J 50:338–344

ZEICHENERKLÄRUNG
CONVENTIONAL SIGNS

Staatsgrenzen	—·—·—·—	International Boundaries
Höhen in Meter	1190	Heights in Meters
Trockentäler, Wadis	··············	Intermittent Rivers, Wadies
Wasserfälle	～✕～	Waterfalls
Sümpfe, Überschwemmungsgebiete		Swamp Areas, Flooded Areas
Tundra		Tundra
Salzseen		Salt Lakes
Salzsümpfe		Salt Swamps
Sand- und Dünengebiete		Sandy Deserts
Städte über 1 Million Bewohner	● ■ □	Towns of more than 1,000,000 Inhabitants
Städte von 100 000 bis 1 Million Einwohner	⊙	Towns of 100,000 to 1 Million Inhabitants
Städte, Orte unter 100 000 Bewohner	○	Towns and Villages of less than 100,000 Inhabitants
Hauptstädte	MADRID	Capitals of Countries
Karawanen- und Pilgerwege	– – – –	Caravan Routes
Eisenbahnen	———	Railroads
Kanäle	———	Canals
Flüsse	～～	Rivers

Medizinische Länderkunde/ Geomedical Monograph Series

Beiträge zur geographischen Medizin/Regional Studies in Geographical Medicine. Schriftenreihe der/Series of Monographs of the Heidelberger Akademie der Wissenschaften. Mathematisch-naturwissenschaftliche Klasse. Begründet von/ Founded by: E. Rodenwaldt.

Herausgeber/Editor: **H.J.Jusatz**

The Geomedical Monograph Series is devoted to interdisciplinary studies of countries around the world. Compiled by physicians as well as geographers, these monographs are the result of many years of accumulated knowledge of and experience with the prevalent medical, socioeconomic, and geographic conditions in the countries discussed. The transmission and geographic occurrence of communicable and noncommunicable diseases and the environmental factors influencing them are portrayed in relation to operating geographic conditions. Each volume is directed toward both physicians and geographers, and can serve as a reference for those working in aid programs for developing countries, medical practitioners, economic advisors and travelers.

Volume 3

Äthiopien – Ethiopia

Von/By K. F. Schaller and W. Kuls
Eine geographisch-medizinische Landeskunde
A Geomedical Monograph
Mit einem geographischen Beitrag von/With a Geographic Contribution by W. Kuls
For the English Translation: J. A. Hellen, I. F. Hellen
1972. 64 Bilder, 34 Abbildungen, 7 Karten.
XV, 180 Seiten (In Deutsch und Englisch)
Gebunden DM 68,–
ISBN 3-540-05829-X

"...a readable book as well as a reference manual. The 419 references form an invaluable bibliography. The 64 photographs are of an exceptionally high standard, matched by that of the 7 maps, which include distribution maps of malaria, *Anopheles* mosquitoes, yellow fever, and health institutions... Is is fitting that such a beautiful, breath-taking country, with such energetic and fascinating peoples, should have a reference work of similar quality."

(Tropical Disease Bulletin)

Volume 4
G. E. Ffrench, A. G. Hill

Kuwait

Urban and Medical Ecology – A Geomedical Study
1971. 61 figures, 26 Text figures, 56 tables, 3 maps.
XIII, 124 pages
Cloth DM 58,–
ISBN 3-540-05384-0

Volume 5

Kenya

By H. J. Diesfeld and H. K. Hecklau
A Geomedical Monograph
Translated from the German by J. A. Hellen, I. F. Hellen
1978. 60 photos, 17 figures, 9 map-plates, 55 tables.
XII, 134 pages
Cloth DM 78,–
ISBN 3-540-08729-X

"This book maintains the high standards of accuracy, comprehensiveness of textual and visual information and superb presentation noted in the previous books of the same series. It is another splendid achievement of the authors and publishers, who deserve sincere congratulations not only on the quality of this book but also on its modest price, in relation to its value."

(Tropical Doctor)

Volume 6
C. T. Soh

Korea

A Geomedical Monograph of the Republic of Korea
With Cartographical Contributions of E. Dege
1980. 45 photos, 18 figures, 5 map-plates, 38 tables.
XV, 146 pages
Cloth DM 98,–
ISBN 3-540-09128-9
Distribution rights for Korea: KUMI Trading Co. Ltd., Seoul

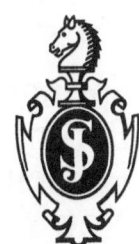

Springer-Verlag
Berlin
Heidelberg
New York

J. C. Frauenthal

Mathematical Modeling in Epidemiology

Universitext
1980. IX, 118 pages
DM 26,–   ISBN 3-540-10328-7

W. R. Hess, P. G. Howell, D. W. Verwoerd

African Swine Fever Virus. Bluetongue Virus

1971. 5 figures. IV, 74 pages
(Virology Monographs, Volume 9)
Cloth DM 29,–   ISBN 3-211-81006-4

D. L. Ingram, L. E. Mount

Man and Animals in Hot Environments

1975. 84 figures, 14 tables. XI, 185 pages
(Topics in Environmental Physiology and Medicine)
Cloth DM 84,–   ISBN 3-540-06865-1

F. Henschen, B. Maegraith

Grundzüge einer historischen und geographischen Pathologie. Pathological Anatomy of Mediterranean and Tropical Diseases

1966. 186 Abbildungen. XXII, 586 Seiten (208 Seiten in Englisch)
(Spezielle pathologische Anatomie, Band 5)
Gebunden DM 160,–
Subskriptionspreis Gebunden DM 128,–
ISBN 3-540-03668-7

R. A. Wever

The Circadian System of Man

Results of Experiments Under Temporal Isolation
1979. 181 figures, 11 tables. XI, 276 pages
(Topics in Environmental Physiology and Medicine)
Cloth DM 102,–   ISBN 3-540-90338-0

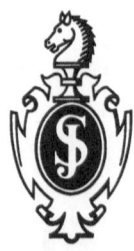

Springer-Verlag
Berlin
Heidelberg
NewYork